T0358950

MR Safety

Editor

ROBERT E. WATSON Jr

MAGNETIC RESONANCE IMAGING CLINICS OF NORTH AMERICA

www.mri.theclinics.com

Consulting Editors
SURESH K. MUKHERJI
LYNNE S. STEINBACH

November 2020 • Volume 28 • Number 4

ELSEVIER

1600 John F. Kennedy Boulevard • Suite 1800 • Philadelphia, Pennsylvania, 19103-2899

http://www.mri.theclinics.com

MRI CLINICS OF NORTH AMERICA Volume 28, Number 4
November 2020 ISSN 1064-9689, ISBN 13: 978-0-323-75938-0

Editor: John Vassallo (j.vassallo@elsevier.com)
Developmental Editor: Kristen Helm

© **2020 Elsevier Inc. All rights reserved.**

This periodical and the individual contributions contained in it are protected under copyright by Elsevier, and the following terms and conditions apply to their use:

Photocopying

Single photocopies of single articles may be made for personal use as allowed by national copyright laws. Permission of the Publisher and payment of a fee is required for all other photocopying, including multiple or systematic copying, copying for advertising or promotional purposes, resale, and all forms of document delivery. Special rates are available for educational institutions that wish to make photocopies for non-profit educational classroom use. For information on how to seek permission visit www.elsevier.com/permissions or call: (+44) 1865 843830 (UK)/ (+1) 215 239 3804 (USA).

Derivative Works

Subscribers may reproduce tables of contents or prepare lists of articles including abstracts for internal circulation within their institutions. Permission of the Publisher is required for resale or distribution outside the institution. Permission of the Publisher is required for all other derivative works, including compilations and translations (please consult www.elsevier.com/permissions).

Electronic Storage or Usage

Permission of the Publisher is required to store or use electronically any material contained in this periodical, including any article or part of an article (please consult www.elsevier.com/permissions). Except as outlined above, no part of this publication may be reproduced, stored in a retrieval system or transmitted in any form or by any means, electronic, mechanical, photocopying, recording or otherwise, without prior written permission of the Publisher.

Notice

No responsibility is assumed by the Publisher for any injury and/or damage to persons or property as a matter of products liability, negligence or otherwise, or from any use or operation of any methods, products, instructions or ideas contained in the material herein. Because of rapid advances in the medical sciences, in particular, independent verification of diagnoses and drug dosages should be made.

Although all advertising material is expected to conform to ethical (medical) standards, inclusion in this publication does not constitute a guarantee or endorsement of the quality or value of such product or of the claims made of it by its manufacturer.

Magnetic Resonance Imaging Clinics of North America (ISSN 1064-9689) is published quarterly by Elsevier Inc., 360 Park Avenue South, New York, NY 10010-1710. Months of issue are February, May, August, and November. Business and Editorial Offices: 1600 John F. Kennedy Blvd., Ste. 1800, Philadelphia, PA 19103-2899. Customer Service Office: 3251 Riverport Lane, Maryland Heights, MO 63043. Periodicals postage paid at New York, NY and additional mailing offices. Subscription prices are $404.00 per year (domestic individuals), $773.00 per year (domestic institutions), $100.00 per year (domestic students/residents), $437.00 per year (Canadian individuals), $1007.00 per year (Canadian institutions), $550.00 per year (international individuals), $1007.00 per year (international institutions), $100.00 per year (Canadian students/residents), and $275.00 per year (international students/residents). International air speed delivery is included in all *Clinics* subscription prices. All prices are subject to change without notice. **POSTMASTER:** Send address changes to *Magnetic Resonance Imaging Clinics*, Elsevier Health Sciences Division, Subscription Customer Service, 3251 Riverport Lane, Maryland Heights, MO 63043. Customer Service (orders, claims, online, change of address): Elsevier Health Sciences Division, Subscription **Customer Service, 3251 Riverport Lane, Maryland Heights, MO 63043. Tel:1-800-654-2452 (U.S. and Canada); 314-447-8871 (outside U.S. and Canada). Fax: 314-447-8029. E-mail: journalscustomerservice-usa@elsevier.com (for print support); journalsonlinesupport-usa@elsevier. com (for online support)**.

Reprints. For copies of 100 or more of articles in this publication, please contact the Commercial Reprints Department, Elsevier Inc., 360 Park Avenue South, New York, NY 10010-1710. Tel.: 212-633-3874; Fax: 212-633-3820; E-mail: reprints@elsevier.com.

Magnetic Resonance Imaging Clinics of North America is covered in the *RSNA Index of Imaging Literature, MEDLINE/PubMed (Index Medicus),* and *EMBASE/Excerpta Medica.*

Contributors

CONSULTING EDITORS

SURESH K. MUKHERJI, MD, MBA, FACR
Clinical Professor, Marian University, Director
of Head and Neck Radiology, ProScan
Imaging, Regional Medical Director, Envision
Physician Services, Carmel, Indiana

LYNNE S. STEINBACH, MD, FACR
Emeritus Professor of Radiology on Full Recall,
Department of Radiology and Biomedical
Imaging, University of California, San
Francisco, San Francisco, California

EDITOR

ROBERT E. WATSON Jr, MD, PhD, MRMD
Neuroradiologist, Department of Radiology,
Mayo Clinic, Rochester, Minnesota

AUTHORS

LOUAI AL-DAYEH, MD, PhD
Boston Scientific Neuromodulation, Valencia,
California

KIMBERLY K. AMRAMI, MD
Department of Radiology, Mayo Clinic,
Rochester, Minnesota

CANDICE A. BOOKWALTER, MD, PhD
Assistant Professor, Department of Radiology,
Mayo Clinic, Rochester, Minnesota

HEIDI A. EDMONSON, PhD
Department of Radiology, Mayo Clinic,
Rochester, Minnesota

ANDREW J. FAGAN, PhD
Department of Radiology, Mayo Clinic,
Rochester, Minnesota

JOEL P. FELMLEE, PhD
Department of Radiology, Mayo Clinic,
Rochester, Minnesota

MATTHEW A. FRICK, MD
Department of Radiology, Mayo Clinic,
Rochester, Minnesota

**TOBIAS BENJAMIN GILK, MArch, MRSO
(MRSC), MRSE (MRSC)**
Senior Vice President, Radiology-Planning,
Kansas City, Missouri; Founder, Gilk Radiology
Consultants, Overland Park, Kansas

MICHAEL N. HOFF, PhD
Department of Radiology, University of
Washington, Seattle, Washington

BHARATHI D. JAGADEESAN, MD
Associate Professor, Radiology, Neurology
and Neurosurgery, University of Minnesota,
Minneapolis, Minnesota

**EMANUEL KANAL, MD, FACR, FISMRM,
MRMD, MRSE**
Chief, Division of Emergency Radiology and
Teleradiology, Director, Magnetic Resonance
Services, Professor of Radiology and
Neuroradiology, Department of Radiology,
University of Pittsburgh Medical Center,
Pittsburgh, Pennsylvania

VERA KIMBRELL, BSRT, R MR FSMRT
MR Clinical Educator, Brigham and Women's
Hospital, Boston, Massachusetts; Chair, SMRT
Safety Committee 2020, Mendon,
Massachusetts

JASON T. LITTLE, MD
Instructor, Department of Radiology, Mayo Clinic, Rochester, Minnesota

JENNIFER S. McDONALD, PhD
Associate Professor, Department of Radiology, Mayo Clinic, Rochester, Minnesota

ROBERT J. McDONALD, MD, PhD
Assistant Professor, Department of Radiology, Mayo Clinic, Rochester, Minnesota

MIZAN RAHMAN, PhD
Boston Scientific Neuromodulation, Valencia, California

JEFFREY ROGG, MD
Medical Director of MRI at Rhode Island Hospital, Associate Professor, Department of Diagnostic Imaging, The Warren Alpert Medical School of Brown University, East Greenwich, Rhode Island

ROGER JASON STAFFORD, PhD
Department of Imaging Physics, The University of Texas MD Anderson Cancer Center, Houston, Texas

MUSSIE TESFALDET, RT
Department of Radiology, University of Washington, Seattle, Washington

ROSS VENOOK, PhD
Boston Scientific Neuromodulation, Valencia, California

JULEE WARREN, RT
Department of Radiology, Mayo Clinic, Rochester, Minnesota

ROBERT E. WATSON Jr, MD, PhD, MRMD
Neuroradiologist, Department of Radiology, Mayo Clinic, Rochester, Minnesota

KIRK M. WELKER, MD
Department of Radiology, Mayo Clinic, Rochester, Minnesota

Contents

Magnetic resonance (MR) imaging–related injuries have continued to occur at an alarming rate during more than 3 decades of use. Persistently reported MR imaging–related injuries are caused by (1) radiofrequency thermal effect burns, (2) bruising from table top and coil-related mechanical injuries, (3) magnetic field–related support equipment malfunction, (4) magnetic field–related projectile trauma, (5) gradient switching noise hearing loss. A cohesive and educated MR imaging community under the guidance of a defined management structure is essential for monitoring and mitigating MR imaging risks. This article offers an approach for decreasing MR imaging–related injury risks.

Although comparatively much younger as a discipline, these early decades of the structure of practice of MR imaging safety have developed in an alarmingly ad hoc manner, particularly when contrasted with contemporary ionizing radiation safety. This absence of structure and metrics for MR imaging safety has impaired the direct safety best practices for the recognizable domains of clinical and operational MR safety. If the built environment of MR imaging is effectively the hardware of the mechanism of health care delivery, then the appropriateness of this hardware to the software (clinical and operational practices) is of great importance.

Conducting magnetic resonance imaging (MRI) safety screening is not a new idea and has developed as a proved method in efforts to ensure patient safety and prevent accidents in the magnetic resonance (MR) environment. A growing number of surgical procedures with implanted medical devices have complicated MR screening and added to the workload of Level 2 personnel. Level 2 staff members are trained to understand and implement screening procedures and should be consulted by all individuals requiring access to the MR environment. All the steps have potential gaps, but as a whole offer efficient and effective tools to alleviate MR-related accidents.

Gadolinium (Gd)-based contrast agents (GBCAs) have revolutionized of MR imaging, enabling physicians to obtain life-saving medical information that often cannot be obtained with unenhanced MR imaging or other imaging modalities. Since regulatory approval in 1988, more than 450 million intravenous GBCA doses have been administered worldwide, with an extremely favorable pharmacologic safety profile. Recent evidence has demonstrated, however, that a small fraction of Gd is retained in human tissues. No direct correlation between Gd retention and clinical effects has been confirmed; however, a subset of patients have attributed various symptoms to GBCA exposure. This review details current knowledge regarding GBCA safety.

MRI is a powerful diagnostic tool with excellent soft tissue contrast that uses nonionizing radiation. These advantages make MRI an appealing modality for imaging the pregnant patient; however, specific risks inherent to the magnetic resonance environment must be considered. MRI may be performed without and/or with intravenous contrast, which adds further fetal considerations. The risks of MRI with and without intravenous contrast are reviewed as they pertain to the pregnant or lactating patient and to the fetus and nursing infant. Relevant issues for gadolinium-based contrast agents and ultrasmall paramagnetic iron oxide particles are reviewed.

Magnetic resonance (MR) imaging relies on a strong static magnetic field in conjunction with careful orchestration of pulsed linear gradient magnetic fields and radiofrequency magnetic fields in order to generate images. The interaction of these fields with patients as well as materials with magnetic or conducting properties can be a source of risk in the MR environment. This article provides a basic review of the physical underpinnings of the primary risks in MR imaging to foster development of intuition with respect to both patient and risk management in the MR environment.

Three dimensionally mapping the relative spatial distributions and magnitudes of the various energy sources used in the MR imaging process for a given MR scanner potentiates an understanding of the relative spatial distributions of the potential risks associated with each of these energies or fields. By systematically analyzing the data for each energy source relative to the location and type of implants, devices, and/or foreign bodies within a specific patient, one can prospectively assess and even begin to quantify the risks of exposing that patient to selected MR scanner hardware for a requested diagnostic study.

New implanted medical devices continue to be made available for treatment of medical conditions. Many recipients can benefit from the diagnostic power of MR imaging. Provisions must be made to determine if these patients can be safely scanned. Metal-containing devices can be considered either MR unsafe or conditional. It is essential that all components of an implanted system are completely and accurately identified, with the most restrictive MR safety condition dictating the scanning approach. MR safety considerations for major classes of implanted devices are discussed, recognizing that there have been reports of serious device-related MR safety incidents.

MR imaging of patients with implanted devices has become common, with conditions for safe scanning defined in MR Conditional labeling of the medical device. This resulted from collaboration among medical device manufacturing, MR imaging scanner manufacturing, and regulatory authority communities. These efforts resulted in engineering testing standards and methods that enable evaluation and certification of devices for safe scanning of patients within prescribed MR imaging scanning conditions. This article provides a practical perspective on test methods that address distinct potential patient hazards. It also provides general guidelines for how a clinician might think about potential hazards, and guidance on common misconceptions.

The arrival of 7T MR imaging into the clinic represents a significant step-change in MR technology. This article describes safety concerns associated with imaging at 7T, including the increased magnetic forces on magnetic objects at 7T and the interaction of the 300 MHz (Larmor) radiofrequency energy with tissue in the body. A dedicated multidisciplinary 7T Safety team should develop safety policies and procedures to address these safety challenges and keep abreast of best practice in the field. The off-label imaging of implanted devices is discussed, and also the need for staff training to deal with complexities of patient handling and image interpretation.

Interventional MR imaging procedures are rapidly growing in number owing to the excellent soft tissue resolution of MR imaging, lack of ionizing radiation, hardware and software advancements, and technical developments in MR imaging-compatible robots, lasers, and ultrasound equipment. The safe operation of an interventional MR imaging system is a complex undertaking, which is only possible with multidisciplinary planning, training, operations and oversight. Safety for both patients and operators is essential for successful operations. Herein, we review the safety concerns, solutions and challenges associated with the operation of a modern interventional MR imaging system.

Multiple factors, including tight patient scheduling, complex electronic medical records, and increasing numbers of implanted devices, increase chances of MR imaging safety event occurrence. Several MR imaging safety incidents are described in this article, including the safety conditions and other factors that contributed to the events. MR imaging safety policy and procedural improvements that address these are also described. Specific new revision points in the American College of Radiology Manual on MR Safety are viewed in the context of these events, with emphasis on how their implementation could reduce probability of similar event recurrence.

MAGNETIC RESONANCE IMAGING CLINICS OF NORTH AMERICA

SERIES OF RELATED INTEREST

Advances in Clinical Radiology
Available at: www.advancesinclinicalradiology.com

Neuroimaging Clinics of North America
Available at: www.neuroimaging.theclinics.com

PET Clinics
Available at: www.pet.theclinics.com

Radiologic Clinics of North America
Available at: www.radiologic.theclinics.com

VISIT THE CLINICS ONLINE!
Access your subscription at:
www.theclinics.com

PROGRAM OBJECTIVE
The goal of Magnetic Resonance Imaging Clinics of North America is to keep practicing physicians up to date with current clinical practice by providing timely articles reviewing the state of the art in patient care.

TARGET AUDIENCE
All practicing physicians and healthcare professionals who provide patient care utilizing findings from Magnetic Resonance Imaging.

LEARNING OBJECTIVES
Upon completion of this activity, participants will be able to:
1. Review safety concerns and considerations associated with various classes of implanted devices, imaging at 7T, GBCA (including Gd retention), and pregnant or lactating patients (as well as the fetus and nursing infant).
2. Discuss risks, improvement to standards of care, and a practical and clinically relevant approach for decreasing MRI related incidents and injuries.
3. Recognize how PEMS improvements can be implemented without meaningful interruption to MRI patient care services as well as a practical perspective on the different test methods that address distinct potential patient hazards.

ACCREDITATION
The Elsevier Office of Continuing Medical Education (EOCME) is accredited by the Accreditation Council for Continuing Medical Education (ACCME) to provide continuing medical education for physicians.

The EOCME designates this journal-based CME activity enduring material for a maximum of 12 *AMA PRA Category 1 Credit*(s)™. Physicians should claim only the credit commensurate with the extent of their participation in the activity.

All other healthcare professionals requesting continuing education credit for this enduring material will be issued a certificate of participation.

DISCLOSURE OF CONFLICTS OF INTEREST
The EOCME assesses conflict of interest with its instructors, faculty, planners, and other individuals who are in a position to control the content of CME activities. All relevant conflicts of interest that are identified are thoroughly vetted by EOCME for fair balance, scientific objectivity, and patient care recommendations. EOCME is committed to providing its learners with CME activities that promote improvements or quality in healthcare and not a specific proprietary business or a commercial interest.

The planning committee, staff, authors and editors listed below have identified no financial relationships or relationships to products or devices they or their spouse/life partner have with commercial interest related to the content of this CME activity:
Kimberly K. Amrami, MD; Candice A. Bookwalter, MD, PhD; Regina Chavous-Gibson, MSN, RN; Heidi A. Edmonson, PhD; Andrew J. Fagan, PhD; Joel P. Felmlee, PhD; Matthew A. Frick, MD; Tobias Benjamin Gilk, MArch, MRSO (MRSC), MRSE (MRSC); Michael N. Hoff, PhD; Bharathi D. Jagadeesan, MD; Emanuel Kanal, MD, FACR, FISMRM, MRMD, MRSE; Vera Kimbrell, BSRT, R MR FSMRT; Pradeep Kuttysankaran; Jason T. Little, MD; Suresh K. Mukherji, MD, MBA, FACR; Jeffrey Rogg, MD; Roger Jason Stafford, PhD; Lynne S. Steinbach, MD, FACR; Mussie Tesfaldet, RT; John Vassallo; Julee Warren, RT; Robert E. Watson Jr, MD, PhD, MRMD; Kirk M. Welker, MD

The planning committee, staff, authors and editors listed below have identified financial relationships or relationships to products or devices they or their spouse/life partner have with commercial interest related to the content of this CME activity:
Louai Al-Dayeh, MD, PhD: employed by Boston Scientific Corporation

Jennifer S. McDonald, PhD: consultant/advisor and research support from General Electiric Company

Robert J. McDonald, MD, PhD: consultant/advisor and research support from General Electiric Company; research support from Bracco Diagnostics Inc.

Mizan Rahman, PhD: employed by Boston Scientific Corporation

Ross Venook, PhD: employed by Boston Scientific Corporation

UNAPPROVED/OFF-LABEL USE DISCLOSURE
The EOCME requires CME faculty to disclose to the participants:
1. When products or procedures being discussed are off-label, unlabelled, experimental, and/or investigational (not US Food and Drug Administration [FDA] approved); and
2. Any limitations on the information presented, such as data that are preliminary or that represent ongoing research, interim analyses, and/or unsupported opinions. Faculty may discuss information about pharmaceutical agents that is outside of FDA-approved labelling. This information is intended solely for CME and is not intended to promote off-label use of these medications. If you have any questions, contact the medical affairs department of the manufacturer for the most recent prescribing information.

TO ENROLL

To enroll in the *Magnetic Resonance Imaging Clinics of North America* Continuing Medical Education program, call customer service at 1-800-654-2452 or sign up online at http://www.theclinics.com/home/cme. The CME program is available to subscribers for an additional annual fee of USD 260.00.

METHOD OF PARTICIPATION

In order to claim credit, participants must complete the following:

1. Complete enrolment as indicated above.
2. Read the activity.
3. Complete the CME Test and Evaluation. Participants must achieve a score of 70% on the test. All CME Tests and Evaluations must be completed online.

CME INQUIRIES/SPECIAL NEEDS

For all CME inquiries or special needs, please contact elsevierCME@elsevier.com.

Foreword
Magnetic Resonance Safety

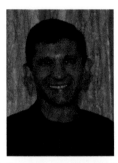

Suresh K. Mukherji, MD, MBA, FACR
Consulting Editor

Radiology is the most technically advanced and innovative medical specialty. Every day I marvel at our capability to create images with radiation, magnets, and "sugar." We have been a victim of our success, and the importance of our specialty has resulted in higher volumes, faster through-puts, different magnet strengths, and new contrast agents. As we struggle to keep up with higher volumes and lower reimbursements and to adapt to an uncertain future, we must always remember that we have the responsibility to maintain a culture of safety for our patients and team members.

This responsibility is especially important in magnetic resonance (MR) imaging and was the inspiration to devote a specific issue to MR safety. I was thrilled when Dr Robert Watson, MD, PhD, MRMD accepted our invitation to guest edit this important issue. The topics are superb and highlight the major issues we face in our daily practice. I would like to personally express my gratitude to all the world-class authors for their outstanding contributions.

Dr Watson has an illustrious career, which includes being Neuroradiology Division Director at the Mayo Clinic and current Chair of both the American Board of MR Safety and the American College of Radiology Safety Committees. I had the privilege of meeting Bob when I was a Visiting Professor at the Mayo Clinic and what impressed me the most was his grace, dignity, and humility. Bob's scholarly accomplishments are only exceeded by his character, and I thank you, Bob, for this wonderful contribution and your collegiality.

Suresh K. Mukherji, MD, MBA, FACR
Clinical Professor, Marian University
Director of Head and Neck Radiology
ProScan Imaging
Regional Medical Director
Envision Physician Services
Carmel, IN, USA

E-mail address:
sureshmukherji@hotmail.com

Magn Reson Imaging Clin N Am 28 (2020) xiii
https://doi.org/10.1016/j.mric.2020.08.004
1064-9689/20/© 2020 Published by Elsevier Inc.

Preface
MR Safety: Coming of Age

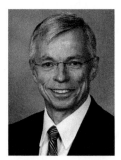

Robert E. Watson Jr, MD, PhD, MRMD
Editor

It has been an honor to serve as guest editor of this issue of *Magnetic Resonance Imaging Clinics of North America* devoted to MR Safety. Increasingly, MR safety as a discipline is truly coming of age, driven by the fine authors included in this issue, as well as many others in the MR community worldwide who understand the importance of "First, do no harm." Regardless of the many technological advances that steadily increase the unparalleled diagnostic power of MR imaging, we are all aware that this same technology can, and has, led to serious injuries and deaths, with common factors being lack of understanding of that technology and/or failure to scrupulously follow well-designed safety processes and procedures each and every time.

A number of factors collectively make maintaining a safe MR environment more challenging in today's practices; among them, ever-more patients and tighter scheduling, our complex electronic systems and environments, increasing use of MR in nonconventional interventional settings, and the ever-increasing numbers of implanted devices in our patients (and, as of this writing, throw COVID-19 into the mix). Reported safety events may be increasing, and while some conclude from this that our practices are increasingly unsafe, I would counter that with the extraordinarily positive steps today in furthering safety in MR. There is an increasing momentum behind embracing a Culture of Safety, and understanding the value of being transparent and sharing MR safety incidents with the intention of the entire MR community learning from them. The American Board of MR Safety now exists, a realization of the vision by Dr Manny Kanal, who understood the

importance of individuals demonstrating tangible knowledge in MR safety, and an organizational structure supporting MR safety comprising a triumvirate of MR Medical Director, MR Safety Expert, and MR Safety Officer. A number of MR safety training courses now exist, led by passionate and extremely knowledgeable MR safety faculty. Manufacturers now exist that produce sensitive ferromagnetic detection equipment, doorway protection devices, and other equipment for safe use in the MR environment. Implant manufacturers devote considerable resources to defining conditions for safe scanning, among other notable examples.

I can't thank our fine authors, all luminaries and experts in their fields, enough for their hard work to produce the top-notch articles that comprise this issue. It is organized such that initial articles by Dr Jeff Rogg, Toby Gilk, and Vera Kimbrell provide overviews of MR safety from the perspective of themes of clinical practice, including considerations of optimal design of MR facilities, and how best to effectively screen patients. Following that, in-depth articles by Dr Bob McDonald and Dr Jennifer McDonald address considerations around gadolinium-based contrast agents, and Dr Jason Little and Dr Candice Bookwalter cover the important topic of MR safety in the context of pregnancy and lactation.

Next, there's an excellent considerably deep dive into the physics of MR safety provided by Dr Jason Stafford. Dr Manny Kanal's article on exciting ground-breaking new technology to help us visualize MR fields and their interaction with implanted devices follows and is followed by an article by MR Safety Expert Dr Heidi Edmonson

Magn Reson Imaging Clin N Am 28 (2020) xv–xvi
https://doi.org/10.1016/j.mric.2020.08.003
1064-9689/20/© 2020 Published by Elsevier Inc.

and me on active implanted electronic devices. Rounding out this section is an important article by Dr Louai Al-Dayeh and colleagues on test methods employed for determining MR conditional status of active implanted devices.

The next section comprises 2 articles addressing MR safety issues in novel environments. The first article on MR safety in 7 T is provided by Dr Andrew Fagan and colleagues and excellently covers the state-of-the-art in MR safety around this game-changing diagnostic tool. The next topic relates to the extremely challenging and variable interventional MR environment, excellently covered by Dr Bharathi Jagadeesan.

A final article, co-authored by Dr Michael Hoff and colleagues, describes several MR safety events, lessons learned from these, and how these relate to updates to the ACR Manual on MR Safety.

To conclude, my sincere thanks go to Dr Suresh Mukherji for inviting me to be part of this rewarding endeavor. Also, sincere thanks to the fine staff at Elsevier, who helped make this a reality, including John Vassallo and Don Mumford. To the authors, heartfelt thanks for sticking with it. And, finally, to you, the readers, thank you for your commitment to MR safety.

Robert E. Watson Jr, MD, PhD, MRMD
Department of Radiology
Mayo Clinic, 200 First Street
Rochester, MN 55905, USA

E-mail address:
watson.robert16@mayo.edu

Key Elements of Clinical Magnetic Resonance Imaging Safety: It Takes a Village

Jeffrey Rogg, MD

KEYWORDS

- MR imaging safety • MR imaging facility management • MR imaging injuries
- MR imaging best practice • MR imaging injury prevention

KEY POINTS

- The most common magnetic resonance (MR) imaging injuries are (1) burns, (2) bruising from table top and coils, (3) equipment malfunction, (4) projectile events, (5) temporary hearing loss.
- Management structure should include (1) MR medical director; (2) MR safety officer; (3) MR safety expert, each with specifically defined duties pertaining to education, policy development, safety management and record keeping. This structure benefits from community-wide best-practice sharing.
- Antennae effects, near-field effects, and e-field loop effects must be considered for mitigation of radiofrequency-related thermal injuries.
- Physical barriers and MR technologist policing for dangerous personnel or equipment supported by policy establishing the sanctity of zone (Z) 3 and Z4 are required. This requirement includes ferromagnetic screening, physical barrier placement when Z4 door is open, labeling of MR-unsafe equipment in Z3, and MR imaging time-out called immediately before transfer of patients between Z3 and Z4.
- Protocols must be established for redundant checks for MR-unsafe or conditional implants. When unknown, review of medical records, radiographs of head/chest/abdomen/pelvis, or computed tomography topogram should be performed.

INTRODUCTION: MAGNETIC RESONANCE IMAGING SAFETY: THE SCOPE OF THE PROBLEM

Magnetic resonance (MR) imaging has been in clinical use for approximately 35 years. Superlative tissue imaging contrast and resulting high sensitivity for detection of disorders with absence of ionizing radiation have led to an exponential growth in diagnostic use. However, the promise of MR imaging as a safe and effective diagnostic imaging tool has come into question, as reported in the lay press, as potentially dangerous to patients, with little institutionalized regulation or oversight compared with radiographs or computed tomography (CT), and where reliable data

reporting of significant injuries or complications is inconsistent. Even at some of the most renowned institutions, major safety events have occurred during the past several years.[1]

Between 2004 and 2009, the US Food and Drug Administration (FDA) reported a 277% increase in the rate of MR imaging–related accidents, far outstripping the 12% increase in MR imaging patient volume during that same time period.[2] Although the exponential growth in reported adverse events has shown some recent evidence of stabilization, significant modality-specific complications continue to occur at an alarmingly high rate (Fig. 1) with few peer-reviewed published reports highlighting or analyzing the scope of the problem.

Department of Diagnostic Imaging, Rhode Island Hospital, Alpert Medical School of Brown University, 593 Eddy Street, Providence, RI 02903, USA
E-mail address: jrogg@lifespan.org

Magn Reson Imaging Clin N Am 28 (2020) 471–479
https://doi.org/10.1016/j.mric.2020.07.001
1064-9689/20/© 2020 Elsevier Inc. All rights reserved.

mri.theclinics.com

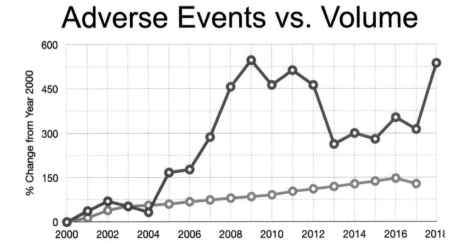

Fig. 1. FDA report of MR imaging–related injuries compared with procedure growth. [a] Interpolated data for years 2008, 2009, 2012, 2013, 2014, and 2015. (*Courtesy of* Tobias Gilk.)

Safety reporting in the United States is largely limited to the FDA Manufacturer and User Facility Device Experience (MAUDE) database, where adverse event reporting is passive, largely relying on voluntary reporting from MR imaging users and patients. Although medical device manufacturers must submit adverse event reports within 30 calendar days when they become aware that a device they market may have caused or contributed to a death or serious injury, self-reported information is often limited or missing in detail, as noted in a recently published MAUDE database review.[3] In this review it was noted that the primary source of patient injury in the MR imaging milieu resulted from (1) mechanical injury–related patient positioning or movement of the MR imaging table top, (2) spatial magnetic field gradient effects resulting in projectile injury or implant malfunction or displacement, (3) radiofrequency (RF) effects causing thermal injury, (4) magnetic field gradient switching effects causing loud noise related to the Lorentz effect or from resulting voltage effects in electrically sensitive sites in the body.

A 3-year review of MR imaging safety incidents in a United Kingdom independent sector provider that operates 70 scanners across the United Kingdom, with nearly 0.5 million patients scanned per year,[4] showed an overall MR imaging safety–related incident rate of 0.05%. Their relative incident rates for specific adverse events, compared with those reported by the National British

Medicines and Healthcare Products Regulatory Agency (MHRA) database, showed projectile incidents accounting for 4.75% (MHRA 7%), burns 1.48% (MHRA 41%), unexpected implant/foreign body 21.5% (MRHA 3%), and acoustic injury 0.89% (MHRA 3%).

This relative rate of MR-related injury is also reflected in the review by Delfino and colleagues[3] of the MAUDE database encompassing the 10-year period from January 1, 2008 through December 31, 2017, which assessed 1568 reported MR imaging events. During this 10-year period, most of the MR imaging–related adverse events resulted from thermal injury (59%), followed by mechanical injuries such as falls, pinch events, or broken ribs related to breast coil use (11%), projectile events (9%), and acoustic injury (6%). This reported relative incidence of MR imaging–related adverse events is consistent with a MAUDE database review from the previous decade (1998–2008), describing a relative incidence of MR imaging–related adverse events of burns (70%), projectiles (10%), implant malfunction (10%), and acoustic injury (4%).[5] Similar relative injury rates were also found in our (Jeffrey Rogg and James Webb, unpublished data, 2020) review of the MAUDE database from December 2009 through December 2019, again showing, in order of occurrence, the greatest MR imaging–related injury risk for burns followed by implant or support equipment malfunction, projectile injury, unexpected foreign body exposure to magnetic field, followed by acoustic injury.

Delfino and colleagues[3] reported 3 deaths specifically related to MR imaging. One patient fatality was attributed to malfunction of an implantable pain pump, where overdischarge of the pharmaceutical occurred. In a second reported death, a field service engineer was crushed by a blower panel that became a projectile while servicing an MR imaging system. A third MR imaging–related fatality resulted when a field engineer sustained a cryogen burn then cardiac arrest while under anesthesia for injury treatment.

Clearly, a review of these injury statistics reflects on the continuing struggle within the radiology community to effectively address MR safety and to protect patients from harm. Despite the commonality through the decades of MR imaging–related safety events, injuries continue to occur with an ongoing and alarming frequency. This article reviews the key elements necessary for helping to create an MR imaging safe environment.

IT TAKES A VILLAGE

Brick-and-mortar design with ironclad policies and procedures, although essential structural components for attempting to ensure MR safety, will not alone suffice without the buy-in of a broad and educated MR imaging patient care community. Members of this hospital-wide community must understand the basic concepts of MR safety and support the common goals and practices for its assurance. The core guiding document for MR imaging safety was initially created by an American College of Radiology (ACR) Blue Ribbon Panel established by the Task Force on Patient Safety of the American College of Radiology and published in 2002 in the *American Journal of Roentgenology*.[6] This document, essential reading for all technologists and physicians, has been expanded and updated through the years (including 2004, 2007, 2013),[7] and most recently in 2020 as an on-line document, titled ACR Manual on MR Safety, maintained by the American College of Radiology.[8]

Even in its earliest form, the 2002 white paper called for the establishment of consistent and thoughtful MR safety policies and practices that included (1) training guidelines and responsibilities for MR technologists, physicians, and support staff; and, (2) defined recommendations for patient screening. The document also reviewed the risks associated with the static magnetic field gradient, RF effects, and time-varying gradients.

The white paper established that a clearly defined management structure was an essential ingredient for ensuring the delivery of MR imaging safety. A recommended structure was later codified in a commentary published in *JMRI* in 2016, reflecting the consensus of the scientific and medical societies in Europe coordinated through the International Society for Magnetic Resonance in Medicine for achieving this purpose.[9] Already practiced at many institutions in the United States, this organizational structure supports the formation of an organic and malleable system for overseeing MR safety that emphasizes self-education, exchange of ideas, and teaching of MR safety. It also supports an organizational structure for managing accountability and providing retrospective assessment when incidents occur, and aids in the prospective planning for an ever-changing clinical environment.

THE KEY COMPONENTS OF THE MAGNETIC RESONANCE SAFETY MANAGEMENT STRUCTURE

The MR medical doctor (MRMD), who is defined as a physician appointed to be responsible for the oversight of 1 or more MR imaging installations with a goal of ensuring (1) the overall safe operation of the MR facilities, which includes issues related to staffing, equipment, and physical structure in order to ensure safe MR examination performance; (2) that the organizational structure also includes an MR safety officer (MRSO) and MR safety expert (MRSE) (their responsibilities are detailed later); (3) that the entity develops, with the MRSO, appropriate and specific policies and procedures pertaining to MR-safe operation; (4) that there is an appropriate system established with the MRSO for ongoing risk assessment, record keeping, and analysis of adverse events, with root cause analysis at the MR facility.

The MRSO, who is typically a senior MR technologist working closely with the MRMD, who is on site. They, or their designee, are available to the MR operators at all times. The MRSO is responsible for (1) ensuring that the policies and procedures for MR imaging safety are routinely performed and enforced; (2) working with the MRMD and MRSE in developing, documenting, and introducing safe working procedures; (3) ensuring that adequate written safety and emergency procedures and instructions are available and issued to all appropriate MR personnel; (4) communicating with and educating MR operators of these policies and procedures; (5) being vigilant of and managing hazards posed within the MR environment as well as taking measures to protect against these hazards; (6) ensuring that all relevant staff groups (ie, nursing medical and environmental services) that may be exposed to MR are educated appropriately as to its potential dangers on a regular basis; (7) consulting with the MRMD/MRSE when advice is required regarding MR safety and reporting back to the MRMD/MRSE any and all MR safety–related issues; (8) ensuring that there is a policy for purchasing, testing, and marking all equipment that will be taken into the MR-related critical areas; (9) providing safety advice on the modification of MR protocols, when necessary in consultation with the MRMD/MRSE.

The MRSE, who is typically an MR physicist, does not need to be available on premises but serves as an advisory resource for the MRMD/MRSO on issues related to MR technology and physics. Although this person is often an MR physicist, others with suitable technical expertise may serve. The MRSE (1) provides advice on engineering, scientific, and administrative aspects of safe use of MR equipment; (2) provides advice on the development and continuing evaluation of the MR environment; (3) provides advice for the development of local rules and procedures regarding MR equipment; (4) provides safety advice on acceptance testing; (5) establishes and maintains links with appropriate district, regional, or professional bodies and reports back to the MRMD/MRSO when appropriate.

In all cases, these individuals are expected to participate in continuing education on MR safety in order to remain abreast of national issues, trends, and standards. National certification for these positions became available in 2016 by a 10-year renewable certificate through the American Board of MR Safety (ABMRS). Although not required by current American professional licensure and certifying organizations, certification by ABMRS is highly recommended to help candidates gain insight into the body of information deemed necessary to adequately assume these important responsibilities. The ABMRS, now with more than 5000 certificate holders, has also inspired an active social networking community with more than 22,000 participants on Facebook (MRI Safety), where ideas, questions, and concerns about MR imaging safety are actively discussed by MR operators throughout the United States and beyond.

The proposed organizational structure and its support for safety responsibility, safety education, policy development, troubleshooting, and problem mitigation can easily extend beyond the confines of any single institutional structure with little effort. In Rhode Island, for example, in addition to our monthly hospital MR staff meetings and safety educational sessions, we coordinate a monthly MR safety meeting that includes our 5 closest hospital neighbors as well as a large private practice radiology group in our community. At these meetings, typically attended by the MRSOs from each entity, we share each other's "dirty laundry" (site of specific incidents may be deidentified if required for medicolegal concerns). This shared safety structure has had significant impact on our ability to identify potential looming safety issues, troubleshoot solutions, and share information regarding new technologies and safety updates. It has also enabled us to develop common best practice and policies within our extended safety community.

PREVENTING THERMAL INJURIES

As described earlier, thermal injuries are consistently the leading cause for MR-related safety incidents. The source of injury is commonly related to effects of the time-varying RF magnetic field, which is primarily concentrated within the central 45 to 60 cm (1.5–2 feet) of the isocenter of the MR bore, varying by MR imaging vendor. Although a detailed description of the physics of RF-related thermal injury is beyond the scope of this article, thermal injury is principally related to (1) RF antennae effects, (2) near-field (electromagnetic field) effects, and (3) e-field loop resonance effects.[10,11] A perusal of the recent 10-year MAUDE database defines several common errors that may lead to patient thermal injuries.

Antennae Effects: Clothing

A frequently cited source of thermal injury is related to absorption of RF energy through the antennae effect when patient clothing or blankets are included within the RF field during an examination that contain metallic electrically conducting material that is often not visible or specifically identified on the fabric label. Unexpected and unpredictable resonance with the transmitted RF can cause significant fabric heating to occur, leading to thermal skin burns or even fires.[12,13] A simple solution to this potential risk is the routine changing of patients' clothing, including underwear, especially when it will be included in the RF field, into facility-supplied safe garments and blankets. For inpatients, this may result in a discussion with purchasing to ensure safe fabrics and that metallic snaps are not present on hospital gowns. For outpatients, we learned that initial patient push-back could be mitigated by supplying surgical scrubs for patients instead of open gowns, and on occasion allowing disabled patients to arrive for their scans in a predetermined, clearly labeled MR-safe garment.

Antenna Effects: Implanted or External Conductors

Another common antennae effect–related thermal injury occurs when implanted or exposed leads (especially when insulated where heat concentrates at the exposed tips) are included in the RF field. External electrocardiogram (ECG) leads,[11] iron-containing tatoos,[14] and metal piercings[15] are also subject to this thermal risk. In such cases, when possible, the conductor should be removed. When not possible, conductor loops should be avoided, a cooling heat sink used, and insulation placed between the conductor and the patient's skin. Implanted conductors require adherence to product documents specifying MR conditions of use. Interrogation for possible lead fracture is typically required to avoid the potential for heating at the fracture site, which often contraindicates MR scanning.

E-Field Loop Effects

Frequent reports of fingertip to lateral thigh and medial thigh burns are present in the MAUDE database. These easily preventable injuries are related to the e-field loop effects caused by RF-induced current deposition in the patient's body. Circulating electrons in a body loop cause heating at sites of conductor narrowing, such as arm to fingertip or fingertip to thigh, where increased resistance at the contact point causes heating leading to thermal skin injury. Pads must be placed between all potential skin contact sites to prevent loop burns from occurring. Similarly, looping of cable or other electrical conductors, especially when in contact with the patient, within the RF field must be avoided.

Near-Field Effects

There are multiple reports in the MAUDE database of thermal injuries, especially in large patients, at sites where the patient's skin contacts the inner wall of the magnet bore. At 1 of our MR locations, a patient received a first-degree burn of his hip during an abdominal MR scan, despite the placement of what our technologist assumed to be an insulating sheet between his skin and the MR plastic wall. Near-field burns likely result from a microwavelike electromagnetic field heating phenomenon resulting from the body part's proximity to the RF transmitting coil. A solution is to ensure the preservation of adequate space between the bore wall and the patient's body. This positioning can typically be achieved by routinely placing MR-specified foam pads at all potential contact points between the patient and the MR imaging bore, creating at least a 1-cm buffer zone.

PREVENTING PROJECTILE INJURIES

The second most common, and perhaps most damaging, MR-related safety hazard may occur when ferromagnetic materials inadvertently enter zone (Z) 4 to become projectiles as they accelerate along the magnetic field gradient to the MR bore. As initially proposed in the 2002 ACR Blue Ribbon Panel, a safe architectural design to limit traffic and material flow in proximity to the MR scanner (**Fig. 2**) can help to mitigate this risk.

In this design, partitions exist between areas accessible to the public (Z1) and the area where unscreened patients, their families, and MR-related personnel have access (Z2). Z2 often also accommodates changing rooms, patient lockers, and prep areas. Z2 is separated from the area outside of the MR imaging scanner rooms (Z3). Z3 has strictly restricted access by a physical barrier and is monitored by the MR imaging technologists, ensuring that all patients, personnel, and materials remaining in Z3 are carefully regulated and conditional or safe to enter the MR scanner room Z4. A door exists between Z3 and Z4. No admittance to Z4 should be permitted without specified personnel training and/or screening. Screening of all patients, family members, or other non-MR personnel must be performed by questionnaire, filled out initially by the person gaining access, and then reviewed verbally a second time by the MR imaging technologist. When necessary, because of inadequate history, review of appropriate prior imaging studies, or performance of radiographs to exclude implanted devices is required. At our institution, in the absence of clear history, visual inspection of the patient is followed by performance of radiographs of the head, chest (including shoulders and upper arms), and abdomen/pelvis (including upper thighs) to exclude the presence of potentially MR-unsafe or conditional implanted devices. For our emergent patients with stroke, we have instituted the practice of performing a whole-body low-radiation topogram at the time of all urgent large vessel occlusion CT/CT angiography examinations, for the potential of follow-up emergent rapid MR imaging examinations.

All hospital inpatients are transferred in Z2 onto an MR imaging safe stretcher with new MR-provided sheets and blankets to reduce the risk of camouflaged foreign bodies entering the room. In addition, all patients are screened with a handheld ferromagnetic detector, with focused investigation of any positive readings before admittance.

Despite these efforts, and acknowledgment of the certainty of human error, we have included 3

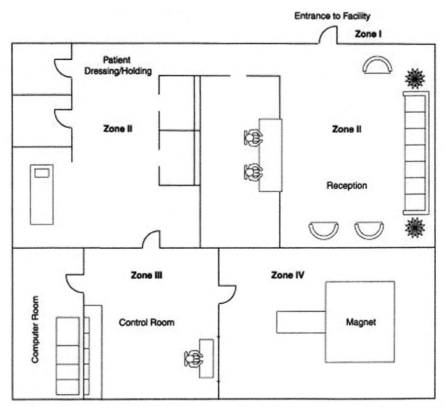

Fig. 2. MR imaging architectural design showing Z1 to Z4, which reduces the potential for unsafe MR imaging materials to enter the scanner room (Z4). (*From* https://www.acr.org/Clinical-Resources/Radiology-Safety/MR-Safety; with permission.)

additional safety safeguards to prevent hazardous penetration of Z4. These solutions were developed by consensus of our Statewide MR Safety Group and then adopted by our 6 participating hospitals and outpatient practice.

Magnetic Resonance Time-Out

Following a near miss involving an MR-unsafe intravenous pole that migrated into Z4 when a patient became unstable in Z3 during transition to Z4, causing failure of our technologist and accompanying nursing staff to follow through on expected transfer to an MR conditional pole, we instituted an MR time-out policy. Similar in scope to operating room side/site time-out safety policy, we perform a full stop in Z3 before moving to Z4 for all emergency department patients, sedated patients, or hospital inpatients, during which time the MR technologist and a second technologist or technical assistant perform a spoken review of the integrity of the screening process. This review includes assurance of the complete and accurate review of safety form, review of adequate ferromagnetic screening performance, and a final visual review and verbal assurance of the safety of

all accompanying devices and personnel before patient transfer. This review is followed by documentation that the process occurred and signature by the supervising MR technologist. Statewide acceptance and compliance with this policy, initiated in January 2018, has been unanimous and has resulted in several catches. This full stop and final check procedure has been adopted and published in the ACR guidance document update for 2020.[8]

Physical Safety Barrier in Front of Open Zone 4 Door

Following an event in which an anesthesiologist's forceps clamp launched from his scrubs into the magnet bore when he entered Z4 while a technologist was in the room setting up for the next patient, we initiated the policy of requiring a safety strap (physical barrier) in front of all Z4 open doors (**Fig. 3**). This policy has also been adopted in the ACR guidance document update 2019, which states that the entry to Z4 should be closed except when it must be open for patient care or room maintenance. During the times that the door must remain open, a caution barrier is

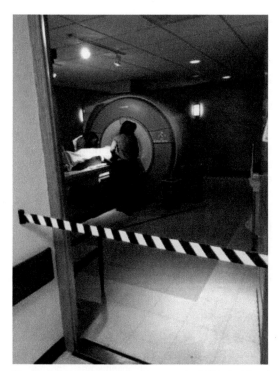

Fig. 3. Retractable safety strap used at Rhode Island Hospital to prevent Z4 room entry when scanner door is open for patient care.

recommended at the entry to Z4 to inhibit unintended entry of personnel or materials. We have also initiated a policy that prohibits the nonemergent entry of all but the supervising MR technologist into Z4 while a patient is in the bore of the magnet. When essential material or personnel must enter Z4 while a scan is underway, the supervising MR technologist removes the patient from the magnet bore before material or personnel entry. The initiation of this policy serves as a further check to help prevent catastrophic patient projectile-related injuries.

Also adopted by our participating sites is a policy stating that all non-MR conditional devices that must remain in Z3 for patient support during scanning are brightly tagged as MR unsafe. We also require all personnel remaining in Z3 during a patient examination to be screened, both verbally and by ferromagnetic detector, for approval for Z4 entry if required for urgent patient care.

IMPLANT MALFUNCTION

Careful screening for the presence of biomedical implants, materials, and devices must be performed in all patients as clearly stated in all previous ACR guidance documents on MR safety at least twice. When the existence of an implant is not known, review of the electronic medical record and/or prior imaging is needed to ascertain the presence of potentially dangerous devices.

As previously stated, at our institution when device implantation is unknown, we routinely obtain 2-view radiographs of the skull and upper neck to rule out implanted aneurysm clip or other wires or devices, single-view chest radiograph to rule out abandoned ECG leads, and single-view kidney, ureter, and bladder, including pelvis (to lesser trochanters), to rule out abandoned neurostimulator or other implants.

When an implant is encountered, safety analysis must include consideration of the ferromagnetic properties, location in the body in relation to sensitive structures, fixation, size, and mass. The device's function and potential alteration in function caused by exposure to the RF, gradient, and magnetic field must all be considered in relation to MR field strength, expected location relative to transmitted RF, and specific absorption rate (SAR). Useful databases that may be routinely searched for device safety and conditions of use are available through device manufacturers and collated at MRISafety.com and www.magresource.com. The identification and safety characteristics of all devices must be clearly marked by primary source verification. Recollection of implanted device identity should not be accepted, nor does the prior safe scanning of a device prove its safety.

As stated earlier, we benefit through the existence of an educated safety management structure where it is the role of the MRSO and MRMD in cooperation with the MRSE to assess the risk and benefit of patient scanning when not clearly defined. The MRSO also works in cooperation with the MRMD to ensure that scan parameters are in accord with published device parameters.

ACOUSTIC INJURY

Acoustic injuries may occur because of the Lorentz effect from the displacement of the magnetic gradients within their casing perpendicular to the B0 field and direction of current flow. The noise level depends on the gradient amplitude and rate of change for a scanning sequence and is affected by slice thickness, field of view, repetition time, and echo time. The FDA requires that MR operators provide hearing protection for acoustic noise greater than 99 dB,[15] and the Occupational Safety and Health Administration permits a daily exposure limit of 90 dB.[16] Typically, foam polyvinyl chloride ear plugs provide up to approximately 29-dB noise reduction, whereas headphones (Siemens Medical, Ehrlanger, Germany) provide approximately 14-dB noise reduction. Because a

1.5-T Aera has an estimated maximum 101.5 dB, standard ear plugs are typically an adequate solution for potential acoustic injury. However, at 3 T (Siemens Verio), the estimated typical scanning acoustic levels can reach more than 115 dB. In a recent study, 26 healthy volunteers were scanned at 3 T for 51 minutes using T1 three-dimensional gradient-recalled echo, T-2 fast spin echo, diffusion tensor imaging, T2*, and blood oxygenation level–dependent imaging sequences. Measured mean exposure was 118 to 123 dBA (A-weighted decibels).[17] The subjects experienced significant increased mean hearing threshold shift of 5.0 to 10 dB immediately after MR compared with baseline, which returned to baseline at 25 days in all cases. However, guarantee of hearing recovery is not assured for all patients.

At our institution, hearing protection is provided at 3 T by using a combination of foam ear plugs in conjunction with headphones, affording combined noise reduction of approximately 43 dB. However, a common complaint with this solution is patient difficulty in hearing technologist instructions during the examination through the earplugs. We have recently adopted the use of the MagnaCoil protective hearing device (www.magnacoustics. com), providing 30-dB hearing protection while enabling the transmission of music and technologist instructions. When patients refuse to comply with the use of provided acoustic noise injury prevention devices, we educate and inform them of their risk for experiencing at least temporary hearing loss, especially at 3 T. Following this discussion, most patients do comply. In the rare circumstance where patients continue to refuse hearing protection, the conversation is documented and attempt is made, when possible, to perform the examination at 1.5 T.

SUMMARY

MR imaging has been providing lifesaving diagnostic capability for more than 35 years, but it remains a potentially dangerous tool if not properly managed and regulated. Reviews of large national and international databases through the decades of MR use focus on the persistent and malicious recurrence of MR morbidity related to thermal injuries, projectile injuries, equipment/device malfunction, and acoustic injury.

It takes a village of dedicated and educated MR imaging professionals, organized into a proactively attentive and responsive structure, to attempt to best ensure MR imaging safety. This organizational structure at its best must remain educated and connected locally and nationally so that it can best develop, initiate, monitor, and share enthusiastic adherence to best practices.

Vigilant focus on the dangers of RF transmission effects on thermal injuries, spatial magnetic field gradient effects on projectile injuries and equipment malfunction, and gradient switching effects on voltage induction and acoustic injuries is essential.

This article offers the author's practical experience and advice for attempting to mitigate these hazards, recognizing that human error can at times overwhelm all barriers, requiring adherence to shared responsibility and responsive management.

DISCLOSURE

The author has no commercial or financial conflicts of interest or significant funding sources relevant to this submission.

REFERENCES

1. Kowalczyk L. MRIs carry rare—but very real—hazards. Boston Globe; 2017. p. 8.
2. Rise in MRI accidents highlights need for magnet safety. Available at: AuntMinnie.com https://www. auntminnie.com/index.aspx?sec=sup&sub=mri& pag=dis&ItemID=86898. Accessed February 1, 2020.
3. Delfino JG, Krainak DM, Flesher SA, et al. MRI-related FDA adverse event reports: A 10-yr review. Med Phys 2019;46(12):5562–71.
4. Hudson D, Jones AP. A 3-year review of MRI safety incidents within a UK independent sector provider of diagnostic services. Microbiologyopen 2019;1(1). bjro.20180006.
5. Joint Commission on Accreditation of Healthcare Organizations, USA. Preventing accidents and injuries in the MRI suite. Sentinel Event Alert 2008;38: 1–3. Available at: https://www.ncbi.nlm.nih.gov/ pubmed/18389573.
6. Kanal E, Borgstede JP, James Barkovich A, et al. American College of Radiology White Paper on MR Safety. Am J Roentgenol 2002;178(6):1335–47.
7. Expert Panel on MR Safety, Kanal E, Barkovich AJ, Bell C, et al. ACR guidance document on MR safe practices: 2013. J Magn Reson Imaging 2013; 37(3):501–30.
8. ACR Committee on MR Safety, Greenberg TD, Hoff MN, Gilk TB, et al. ACR Manual on MR Safety, Version 1.0 2020 American College of Radiology (ACR). Available at: https://www.acr.org/-/media/ ACR/Files/Radiology-Safety/MR-Safety/Manual-on-MR-Safety.pdf.
9. Calamante F, Ittermann B, Kanal E, et al, Inter-Society Working Group on MR Safety. Recommended responsibilities for management of MR safety. J Magn Reson Imaging 2016;44(5):1067–9.

10. Shellock FG. Radiofrequency energy-induced heating during MR procedures: a review. J Magn Reson Imaging 2000;12(1):30–6.

11. Dempsey MF, Condon B. Thermal injuries associated with MRI. Clin Radiol 2001;56(6):457–65.

12. Pietryga JA, Fonder MA, Rogg JM, et al. Invisible metallic microfiber in clothing presents unrecognized MRI risk for cutaneous burn. AJNR Am J Neuroradiol 2013;34(5):E47–50.

13. Bertrand A, Brunel S, Habert M-O, et al. A new fire hazard for mr imaging systems: blankets—case report. Radiology 2018;286(2):568–70.

14. Kreidstein ML, Giguere D, Freiberg A. MRI interaction with tattoo pigments: case report, pathophysiology, and management. Plast Reconstr Surg 1997;

99(6):1717–20. Available at: https://www.ncbi.nlm.nih.gov/pubmed/9145144.

15. Tsai LL, Grant AK, Mortele KJ, et al. A practical guide to MR imaging safety: what radiologists need to know. Radiographics 2015;35(6): 1722–37.

16. Safety and Health Topics | Occupational Noise Exposure | Occupational Safety and Health Administration. 2019. Available at: https://www.osha.gov/SLTC/noisehearingconservation. Accessed February 1, 2020.

17. Jin C, Li H, Li X, et al. Temporary hearing threshold shift in healthy volunteers with hearing protection caused by acoustic noise exposure during 3-T multisequence MR neuroimaging. Radiology 2018; 286(2):602–8.

MR Imaging Safety
Siting and Zoning Considerations

Tobias Benjamin Gilk, MArch, MRSO (MRSC), MRSE (MRSC)[a,b,*]

KEYWORDS

- MR imaging • Safety • Zones • Standards • Practice • Physical environment • Construction
- Renovation

KEY POINTS

- In the past 20 years, MR imaging seems to have steadily produced increasing risk of harm. By contrast, safety initiatives have substantially reduced risk of harm from ionizing radiation usage in diagnostic settings.
- MR imaging safety, as an initiative, has suffered from the absence of formal standards of training or implementation.
- Physical environment MR safety (PEMS) has a significant potentiating capability for clinical and operational safety practices, when effectively integrated. When executed poorly, PEMS initiatives can actively undermine clinical and operational safety practices.
- Although several PEMS initiatives are only practical as a part of a major capital project, many PEMS improvements can be implemented without meaningful interruption to MR imaging patient care services.

INTRODUCTION/BACKGROUND

MR imaging safety, as a discipline, has been poorly formed in practice. With neither radiologists nor MR imaging technologists having formal curriculum in MR imaging safety as a part of their professional education, and with scant licensure or accreditation standard requirements for MR imaging safety that directly combat the sources of MR imaging harm, the structure and practice of MR imaging safety has developed in an alarmingly ad hoc manner, particularly when contrasted with contemporary practices for ionizing radiation safety. In this regard, MR imaging safety has become a victim of its own marketing.

In the past decade, alone, the stochastic risk from diagnostic exposure to ionizing radiation has fallen significantly due to concerted safety efforts on multiple fronts, although very small numbers of deterministic radiation burns continue to occur. It seems that the improvements in radiograph-based imaging technology coupled with practice changes inspired by programs such as "Image Gently" and "Image Wisely" have made marked improvements in the safety of diagnostic modalities that use ionizing radiation.

By contrast, technological improvements in MR imaging over the past 20 years have largely increased risk concerns (eg, more powerful magnetic fields, greater radiofrequency (RF) power, increased slew rates), and there have been no comparable public awareness campaigns for MR imaging to identify or reduce risks or to better report the adverse events that do occur. In this timeframe, MR imaging–classified adverse event report rates to the US Food and Drug Administration (FDA) have accelerated faster than the number of examinations performed.[1] Said plainly, the data suggest that, unlike diagnostic radiography, we are injuring more MR imaging patients today than we were 20 years ago (**Fig. 1**).

When we adjust our focus from the macro to the individual practitioner, we see enormous variability

[a] Radiology-Planning, Kansas City, MO, USA; [b] Gilk Radiology Consultants, PO Box 26466, Overland Park, KS 66225, USA
* Corresponding author. Gilk Radiology Consultants, PO Box 26466, Overland Park, KS 66225.
E-mail address: TGilk@MRIpatientsafety.com
Twitter: @tobiasgilk (T.B.G.)

Magn Reson Imaging Clin N Am 28 (2020) 481–488
https://doi.org/10.1016/j.mric.2020.07.006
1064-9689/20/© 2020 Elsevier Inc. All rights reserved.

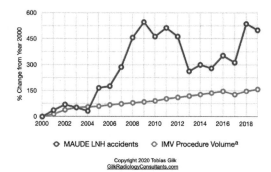

Fig. 1. Chart comparing change in MR imaging total procedure volume versus change in reported MR imaging adverse events from the year 2000 as baseline. [a] Interpolated data for years 2008, 2009, 2012, 2013, 2014, and 2015. (*Courtesy of* T. Gilk, M.Arch., Kansas City, MO.)

in the nature of MR imaging safety training and protections. Contemporary MR imaging safety practices often echo the parable of the 3 blind men who come across an elephant for the first time: each man touching a different part of the elephant and describing the nature of the whole animal based on the part he is touching. In the absence of a formal structure, each of us is free to (erroneously) presume that our own individual perception is both typical and complete. The myth of "the safe modality" inhibits a broader understanding of MR imaging safety risks and the effectiveness of existing practices to effectively manage those risks.

The areas of MR imaging safety that are more typically related to daily practice are those that pertain to operations and clinical decision-making. These areas of practice, while perhaps still lagging behind established best practices, are more familiar and accessible to MR imaging providers and practitioners. Physical environment MR safety (PEMS), by contrast, is substantially dissociated from the daily realm of health care administrators, radiologists, and technologists. But if the built environment of MR imaging (or any health care service) is effectively the hardware of the mechanism of health care delivery, then the appropriateness of this hardware to the software (clinical and operational practices) is of great importance.

PHYSICAL ENVIRONMENT MR SAFETY EXISTING LITERATURE

Although a healthy (and growing) body of MR imaging safety practice literature exists, it largely formally resides in the realm of recommended best practices and not standards. Even omnibus MR imaging safety publications such as the 2020

American College of Radiology (ACR) Manual on MR Safety[2] are presented largely as an anthology of discreet best practice policies and not as a formal structure for MR imaging safety, nor as the ACR's own standards for operation of an ACR-accredited MR imaging provider.[3,4]

Within the realm of physical environment safety for MR, from the AAPM Report 20, to the original 4 Zone model from the ACR, to the Sentinel Event Alert #38 from the Joint Commission (TJC), recommendations for PEMS safety have existed, in one form or another, since 1986.[5–7] In the 2010 edition of the Facilities Guidelines Institute (FGI) Guidelines for Design and Construction of Health Care Facilities, the 4 Zone model became a requirement for the many adopting jurisdictions that use FGI as a health care design standard, although this applied only prospectively to new or renovated facilities.[8] In the Joint Commission's 2015 Diagnostic Imaging Standard, TJC adopted language substantially similar to that of the ACR's 4 Zone model (and yet, TJC's language is significantly less specific).[9] As an accreditation standard, this requirement applies retroactively to even existing MR imaging facilities within Joint Commission accredited sites. The 2018 US Veteran Health Authority Directive 1105.05 on MR safety similarly requires the implementation of the 4 Zone model and further requires line-of-sight and situational awareness as elements of MR imaging suite design and construction.[10]

Because of differences in equipment, patient populations, and clinical needs, PEMS is not well served to copy-and-paste layouts and so it is understandable that the existing standards tend to be rather abstract in their stated requirements. There are infinite design permutations of a 4 Zone concept that can be (should be) tailored to the particular volume, acuity, intervention, and procedural requirements of an individual provider. Simply providing a 4 Zone model, in and of itself, is no assurance of the appropriateness or suitability of a design to the particular operational needs of a given MR imaging provider.

AIMS OF THIS PAPER

This paper works within a formal set of 3 categorical classifications of MR imaging safety practices (clinical MR imaging safety, operational MR imaging safety, and PEMS), which, together, represent a functionally comprehensive structure for thinking of MR imaging safety. From this structure, this paper explores the role that PEMS plays within the comprehensive MR imaging safety structure, the nature of PEMS risks and interventions, and the importance of PEMS considerations. In the end, the goal is that the reader appreciates both the necessity and insufficiency of contemporary PEMS licensure and accreditation standards and how opportunities for improvements to physical environment safety within the MR suite should be identified and carefully planned for.

DISCUSSION

Looking just at MR imaging–classified injuries within the FDA's Manufacturer and User Facility Device Experience database (FDA product code LNH), we see that the most commonly identified MR imaging injuries are, in descending order, burns, projectiles, and hearing damage.[11,12] Substantial prevention of these 3 most frequently reported MR imaging device injuries is possible through existing best practices.[13] These best practices can be categorized as clinical (eg, obtaining complete patient clinical history to identify potential contraindications), operational (eg, providing appropriate padding to reduce burn potential), and physical environment (eg, maintaining access controls to prevent unscreened persons/equipment from entering controlled access regions of the MR imaging suite).

All 3 categorical classifications of MR imaging safety interventions—clinical, operational, and physical environment—are necessary, and prevention of any adverse event type often depends on the successful interrelation of prevention strategies among all three. Effective clinical screening of persons is inhibited in the absence of acoustically private areas to review screening forms. Physical screening of persons is inhibited in the absence of appropriate changing areas, belongings storage, and screening ferromagnetic detection. Proper segregation of screened from unscreened persons is inhibited when there are not effective segregated subwaiting areas and appropriate access controls for the zones. The degree to which operational, clinical, and physical environment MR safety are entangled and mutually supporting cannot be overstated. The benefits of rigorous adherence to operational and clinical

safety best practices will be substantially undermined in a physical environment that is not similarly prepared to support those practices and mitigate the risks inherent to MR.

PHYSICAL ENVIRONMENT MR SAFETY INTERVENTIONS PREVENTING ACCESS OF UNSCREENED INDIVIDUALS

The use of suite diagrams/floor plans has supported a misconception that the 4 Zone model maps ascribe designations to individual rooms or functions. Although designating zones by rooms is the practical implication, zoning (and the resulting access control implications) is the result of risk designations. Zone 4, the MR imaging scanner room, is the only room that has a defined zone (by virtue of the presence of the MR imaging scanner with direct, unfettered access from within the room). All other zones are defined by their presence of MR imaging physical hazards or potential access to regions of MR imaging physical hazard (**Fig. 2**).

The MR imaging control room is often (mis-)understood to be, by definition, a Zone 3 space. It can be a Zone 3 space if either of the 2 risk conditions are met: free physical access into the MR imaging scanner room (Zone 4) or an MR imaging physical hazard is present (eg, static magnetic field strength of 5 Gauss/0.5 mT or greater). If there is no MR imaging physical hazard in the control room, and the door to the MR imaging scanner room is physically locked, in that moment the control room is technically not a Zone 3 area, although from a functional standpoint it is prudent in most instances to treat it as a persistent Zone 3. The understanding of Zoning based on risk is particularly important as Interventional and intraoperative MR grows, with shifting patterns of usage and access, depending on varied clinical demands. Dynamic MR environments, where MR scanners may move between rooms, may require dynamic functional Zone definitions established based on varying risk factors.

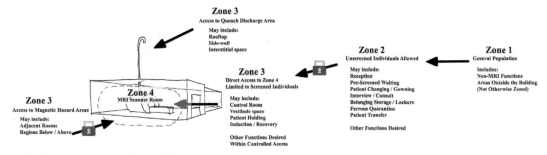

Fig. 2. Risk conditions defining MR imaging Zones.

Because of both the persistence of MR imaging static magnetic field risks in most of the MR imaging sites and the casual imperceptibility of static magnetic fields, it is appropriate to compare the clandestine nature of MR imaging risks with those of radioactive materials; both are devoid of smell, taste, or overt physical sensation. As with a hot laboratory or cyclotron facility's physical restrictions to protect against inadvertent radiation exposure, similar care must be taken with MR imaging facilities to ensure that individuals are not permitted independent access to areas with magnetic field hazards, and this includes facility personnel who may be accustomed to wide-ranging access (eg, maintenance, housekeeping, security, senior management). For example, the 5 G line may cross substantially into an adjacent equipment room, posing a potential risk to individuals with implanted devices that unwittingly enter this space, particularly if there is no clear marking and delineation that this space is technically Zone 3. Access controls, strictly linked to contemporary clinical screening and appropriate safety training, must be rigorously enforced. Increasingly it is the expectation to take the controlled access portions of the MR imaging suite off of facility-level master key access programs and—as with a hot laboratory—tightly control the individuals to whom free access is granted, often tying it to document completion of MR safety training.

Within the MR imaging suite it is wise for the layout to permit the MR technologist/radiographer to have commanding situational awareness from the operator's console. This should include line-of-sight into the MR imaging scanner room with a clear view of a patient inside the scanner, the entrance into the MR imaging scanner room, and entry into the control area. In hospital settings where higher acuity patients are scanned via MR, or where sedation/anesthesia are used, additional consideration should be given to facility layouts to provide observation capabilities for patients who may be temporarily held, undergoing preexamination preparation or postexamination recovery within the MR imaging suite. As such, there should be accommodations made at the planning stages to have, for example, availability of piped-in medical gases within Zone 3 and/or Zone 4.

PHYSICAL ENVIRONMENT MR SAFETY INTERVENTIONS FOR UNSCREENED OBJECTS

Although MR imaging hazards related to either RF magnetic fields or time-varying gradient exposures occur only during an active MR examination, the static magnetic field risks are omnipresent ("the magnet is always on"). One powerful strategy to reduce the associated risk of projectile accidents is to strive to eliminate any and all equipment and materiel that contain ferrous materials or components. Although 100% elimination of ferrous materials may not be possible, dedicated efforts to creating ferrous-free working environments, particularly when used in concert with ferromagnetic detection screening, can markedly reduce the risk factors for projectile accidents.

Ferromagnetic detection (FMD) systems are devices with excellent sensitivity and specificity developed to identify the presence of magnetic or magnetizable materials that may be projectile hazards in proximity to the MR imaging scanner. Required in many places with new MR imaging equipment installations or MR imaging suite construction, FMDs have, in a relatively modest time-frame, become standard within many regulatory or accreditation regimes.[7,14,15]

FMD systems are most typically deployed in 2 different locations, with different screening objectives. Screener-type systems are frequently placed within Zone 2, with patient changing/gowning functions and patient-belonging lockers. The use of screener-type FMDs provides a quality-control validation, particularly when a patient has been changed into MR safe scrubs or gown, as to whether a patient truly did put away all of their belongings that ought not proceed to the MR imaging scanner room (eg, cell phone, money clip, "lucky" pocketknife, firearm). In contrast, doorway-type systems are frequently placed at the entry door into Zone 4. These are intended not only to help catch anything that a patient may have picked up following Zone 2 screening, as well as to provide a measure of screening for staff, visitors, contractors, vendors, and equipment that may be approaching the MR imaging scanner room with the intent to enter. Doorway entry systems may also assist with accreditation compliance criteria related to effective screening of individuals before entering Zone 4.

It is worth noting that FMD products are available in various configurations, facilitating many different siting options. Of all the various siting options, it is strongly recommended to not place an FMD inside the entrance to Zone 4 (on the MR imaging scanner room side of a doorway). Space permitting, doorway FMD systems should be placed shortly before the doorway into Zone 4, with a designated "taxiway" approaching the door that is as clear as possible of extraneous materiel. This taxiway can also be a functional space for any time-out procedures and final clearances before entering the MR imaging scanner room.

PHYSICAL ENVIRONMENT MR SAFETY INTERVENTIONS FOR KNOWN FERROMAGNETIC/MR CONDITIONALLY LIMITED OBJECTS

Notwithstanding efforts toward a ferrous-free working area, many pieces of equipment intended for use in the MR imaging scanner room will have ferromagnetic components and have static magnetic field conditions for safe usage. For equipment such as MR Conditional anesthesia machines, infusion pumps, respirators, biopsy devices, and contrast injectors, specific static magnetic field and spatial field gradient limitations may exist for safe and effective use.

Two recommendations for addressing magnetic field conditions within Zone 4 are to provide an indication on the flooring of the MR imaging scanner room that shows the boundary location for the governing safety indicator (ie, static magnetic field strength or spatial field gradient) and tether points to limit the movement of equipment within the room to areas outside of the boundary areas.

Floor markings can be in the form of a change in flooring material (changing color, or pattern, or texture) at the boundary, creating an alternate appearance immediately around the MR imaging scanner or a line or closely spaced series of points around the MR imaging scanner. With multiple pieces of MR Conditional equipment with different static field conditions, it is recommended to provide a single boundary based on the most restrictive MR Conditional piece of equipment, instead of multiple boundaries for different pieces of equipment, which may become confusing to staff.

Although floor markings are useful visual cues, often it is very easy to move rolling equipment beyond the defined safety boundary.[16] Sites may also wish to consider tether points in the cabinets, wall, or floor of their MR imaging scanner room such that movable equipment is prevented from crossing safety boundaries within the room. Please take note, however, that retrofitting anchors for tether points, particularly in floors or walls, has the potential to damage RF shield enclosures. Only undertake retrofit installations into floors or walls with the guidance and approval of your RF shield vendor. Any construction activities within an MR imaging scanning room with an at-field MR imaging scanner, including the modification of cabinetry, should only be undertaken with great care and attention to safety (**Fig. 3**).

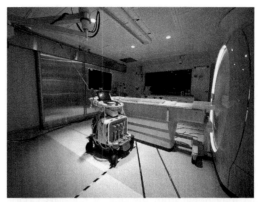

Fig. 3. Tethering of mobile MR imaging unsafe equipment in Zone 4 in interventional MR imaging suite. Note the fixed-length cable tether system that limits movement of the ultrasound system to the (caution) yellow and black striped floor markings at a distance from the magnet. The yellow and black marking matches that on the ultrasound system chassis. The red line marks 300 Gauss; the blue line marks 100 Gauss. (*Courtesy of* Dr. K. Gorny, Mayo Clinic, Rochester, MN.)

For sites that use non-MR Conditional medication pumps or other equipment serving the patient from within the control room, you may wish to consider tether points for non-MR Conditional equipment near the waveguide simply so that the presence of the equipment in the control area does not imply that it is appropriate to bring into the MR imaging scanner room. Consider as well the size, type, and location of the waveguides, whether door jamb type that do not require disconnecting tubing or through-wall type that do.

Within the MR imaging suite, it is also wise to consider the inclusion of dedicated transfer areas, within Zone 2 or Zone 3, where patients on conventional wheelchairs or gurneys can be moved over to MR Conditional transports. Consider also dedicated "quarantine" closets where known ferromagnetic materials (eg, wheelchairs, oxygen cylinders, unsafe medication pumps) may be sequestered to help prevent inadvertent use within the controlled access parts of the MR imaging suite.

PHYSICAL ENVIRONMENT MR SAFETY INTERVENTIONS FOR RADIOFREQUENCY HEATING

Focal heating (thermal injury, burns) is the single-most frequently reported MR imaging adverse event in the United States. The preventions for RF burns pertain to appropriate use of patient preparation, positioning, padding, and the use of MR Conditional patient monitoring equipment.

Although the "last mile" of each of these efforts pertains directly to the actions of the MR technologist, the physical environment plays important roles.

The provision of patient changing and patient belongings storage assists with the patient preparation. The provision of appropriately designed and located storage for bulky positioning aides and patient padding will facilitate their beneficial use. Appropriate storage for patient monitoring equipment and consumables (eg, MR Conditional electrocardiogram leads) also facilitates the appropriate processes to reduce patient harm that may result from the use of non-MR Conditional devices.

In addition, the design of heating, ventilating, and air conditioning (HVAC) systems can help facilitate the maintenance of proper temperature, relative humidity, and airflow within Zone 4, optimizing the shedding of accumulated thermal load of the patient that is the natural bi-product of an MR examination.

PHYSICAL ENVIRONMENT MR SAFETY INTERVENTIONS FOR CRYOGEN SAFETY

Most of the MR imaging scanners make use of liquefied cryogens, typically liquefied helium, to facilitate superconductivity of the primary magnetic field coils. Although rare, under some failure conditions significant quantities of boiled (gaseous) helium could escape into the MR imaging scanner room. The alarming thermal expansion of helium when warming from the temperatures required to keep it in a liquid state ($<-270°$ C) to atmospheric temperatures creates substantial pressure increases.

Many years ago the conventional wisdom had been that doors accessing MR imaging scanner rooms should swing outward from the room, such that a rapid pressure increase within the MR imaging scanner room would push the door open and discharge the accumulating pressure[17] and prevent a "positive pressure entrapment" situation. Changes in RF door technology, however, have made outward-swinging direction of a door ineffective as a safety feature for many more contemporary MR imaging suites. Although some outdated standards persist in recommending (or requiring) outward-swinging doors, these standards do not reflect contemporary best-practice. Outward-swinging doors can impede line of sight viewing of the Zone 4 doorway by the technologist seated at the console if the door swings toward the console.

MR imaging scanner rooms should have positive pressure relief mechanisms, in the form of hatches or, preferably, pressure escape pathways designed as a part of the room's HVAC ductwork systems. With such a system in place, the direction of the swing of the door accessing the MR imaging scanner room is immaterial as a safety protection.

In the event of a cryogen release from the MR imaging scanner (ie, quench), the expanding helium gas should be conveyed through the helium exhaust pipe, more commonly referred to as the quench pipe. The quench pipe effectively serves as a flue or chimney, conveying the escaping helium gas to a safe discharge point. Because of the pressures that develop in quench pipes, and the potential for failure, all MR system manufacturers require annual quench pipe inspections to verify the integrity and patency of quench pathways. In addition, any quench event, or any other event that may have caused building damage at any point along the path of the quench pipe (eg, fire, structural damage, earthquake, water infiltration, etc), should trigger a full repeat inspection of the quench pipe.

At the quench pipe discharge point, an identifiable clear area must be maintained free of operable windows or HVAC air intakes, which might facilitate the reintroduction of helium gas back inside the building. Serviceable equipment in this exclusion zone should be minimized, preferably prohibited, within the clear area. This area should be clearly marked, if not access-restricted, to protect the safety of persons who may be working near the discharge point. MR system manufacturers will provide horizontal and vertical clearance requirements specific to their products, but an exclusion zone of 8 m (25 feet) from the quench pipe discharge point generally accommodates most, if not all, commercial superconducting MR system manufacturer criteria.

Recently, commercial superconducting MR systems have become available that use such small quantities of liquid helium that quench pipes, and specific cryogen safety PEMS preparations to the MR imaging room construction are not recommended by the manufacturer. Nonsuperconducting MR systems, and the new very low-volume cryogen superconducting MR products, will not need these cryogen-specific PEMS interventions. It should be noted, however, that today these very low-volume cryogen systems represent a small proportion of the MR imaging market, and designs for siting these systems may wish to consider that a future replacement magnet may have additional siting requirements for cryogen safety.

TIMELINESS OF PHYSICAL ENVIRONMENT MR SAFETY INTERVENTIONS (CONSTRUCTION, RENOVATION, EQUIPMENT UPGRADES)

Once operational, it is both a financial and patient care burden to interrupt the productivity of an MR imaging suite to implement changes. Unlike operational practices or clinical policies that ought to be regularly reviewed and refined, the physical facility is often "frozen in time," capturing the decisions made in the moment of planning, and not substantially rethought until the next MR imaging installation or replacement (and even then sometimes the proposed solutions are copy-and-paste). Because of the very limited "window of opportunity" for PEMS interventions, and likely long delays between these opportunities, MR imaging providers are well advised to prospectively consider what of their physical environment serves their MR imaging safety needs well and what does not.

With new equipment or new facilities, seize the opportunity to execute on previously planned maps of an idealized workflow and safety experience. With experienced MR imaging or radiology planners, transform that workflow into diagrams of functions and zones and rooms. Anticipate how your clinical and operational needs are likely to change in the next 5 years and ask if your functional diagram readily accommodates those anticipated changes (or what would be necessary to make it do so).

Although many PEMS interventions depend on substantial capital projects, some are easily accomplished between planned major projects with little disruption to clinical operations. Items such as providing an MR imaging suite with MR Conditional support equipment (infusion pumps, anesthesia machines, patient monitoring), installation of FMDs, physical delineation of static magnetic field limitations for MR Conditional equipment or of a time-out area before entry, or even plastic-chain or fabric strap doorway barrier devices can each be implemented rather easily and have positive effects on the physical environment safety of an MR suite. Although some PEMS interventions may be impractical in the absence of a significant renovation, that fact should not dissuade MR imaging providers from analyzing the physical environment safety of their facility and planning the interventions, even if they are comparatively modest, to strengthen the protections against MR imaging accidents and injuries.

ESSENTIAL NATURE OF PHYSICAL ENVIRONMENT MR SAFETY AS A PART OF COMPREHENSIVE MR SAFETY

The more familiar operational and clinical MR safety interventions are often potentiated or subverted as a product of the physical environment in which they take place. MR imaging safety best practices will be made more effective, or possibly functionally impractical, based on the choices that are made with respect to the "bricks and mortar" of an MR imaging provider's facility.

The architect Le Corbusier once stated that the "house is a machine for living," the notion being that we design a space to specifically support the desired activity. The physical spaces we inhabit for delivering patient care are similar; they should be designed and crafted with the specific intent of facilitating the care outcomes we wish to see, including safety. In fact, the more unfamiliar the hazards or objectives, the more care should be dedicated to the crafting of this environment to encourage and facilitate best practice behaviors.

SUMMARY

It is human nature that—as each of the 3 blind men with the elephant—we presume our perspective gives us a reasonably complete view of the problem. However, because of the nature of our daily responsibilities related to MR imaging safety we tend to emphasize more the immediate operational considerations for the technologist and the clinical considerations for the radiologist. PEMS is not typically emphasized in daily responsibilities for anyone in the direct patient care path for MR imaging and as a result may easily be overlooked and poorly acted on at individual facilities. It is for this reason that insightful consideration of PEMS should be elevated by those in the patient care pathways particularly when there are planned MR imaging system upgrades, new system installations, or facility modifications. Successful integration of clinical, operational, and PEMS depends on an effective dialogue among the 3 at points at which each can be tailored to work more effectively with the others.

Clinics care points

- Effective MRI safety must develop clinical MR safety, operational MR safety, and physical environment MR safety (PEMS) in concert.
- PEMS, often divorced from daily staff duties, has the risk of being overlooked or ignored.

- Failure to develop PEMS also has the potential to degrade efficacy of each clinical and operational MR safety.
- While some PEMS interventions are only practical in the context of MRI equipment installation or construction project, many options can be deployed without a major capital project.

DISCLOSURE

Employee, RADIOLOGY-Planning, an architectural design firm specializing in radiology facility design. Owner, Gilk Radiology Consultants, a consulting firm that provides MR imaging safety consultation services.

REFERENCES

1. Mettler F, Mahesh M, Chatfield M, et al. NCRP Report No. 184 – Medical Radiation Exposure of Patients in the United States. 2019. Available at: https://ncrponline.org/shop/reports/report-no-184-medical-radiation-exposure-of-patients-in-the-united-states-2019/. Accessed February 5, 2020.
2. Kanal E, Greenberg T, Hoff M, et al. American College of Radiology ACR manual on MR safety, version 1.0. 2020. Available at: https://www.acr.org/-/media/ACR/Files/Radiology-Safety/MR-Safety/Manual-on-MR-Safety.pdf. Accessed August 25, 2020.
3. Kanal E, Barkovich A, Bell C, et al. American College of Radiology Guidance Document on MR Safe Practices. J Magn Reson Imaging 2013;37:501–30. Available at: https://onlinelibrary.wiley.com/doi/pdf/10.1002/jmri.24011. Accessed February 5, 2020.
4. ACR MR Accreditation Criteria. Available at: https://www.acraccreditation.org/Modalities/MRI. Accessed February 5, 2020.
5. AAPM Report 20 – Site Planning for Magnetic Resonance Imaging Systems. Available at: https://www.aapm.org/pubs/reports/RPT_20.pdf. Accessed February 5, 2020.
6. Kanal E, Borgstede J, Barkovich A, et al. American College of Radiology White Paper on MRI Safety. Am J Roentgenology 2002;178:1335–47. Available at: https://www.ajronline.org/doi/abs/10.2214/ajr.178.6.1781335. Accessed February 5, 2020.
7. Joint Commission Sentinel Event Alert 38: Preventing Accidents and Injuries in the MRI Suite. Available at: https://www.jointcommission.org/en/resources/patient-safety-topics/sentinel-event/sentinel-event-alert-newsletters/sentinel-event-alert-issue-38-preventing-accidents-and-injuries-in-the-mri-suite/. Accessed February 5, 2020.
8. Guidelines for design and construction of health care facilities. St Louis (MO): Facilities Guideline Institute; 2010. Available at: https://fgiguidelines.org/guidelines/2010-edition/purchase/. Accessed February 5, 2020.
9. Joint Commission Hospital Accreditation Program: Diagnostic Imaging Standard. Available at: http://www.jointcommission.org/assets/1/6/HAP-CAH_DiagImag_Prepub_July2015release_20150105.pdf. Accessed February 5, 2020.
10. VHA Directive 1105.05 Magnetic Resonance (MR) Safety. Available at: https://www.va.gov/vhapublications/ViewPublication.asp?pub_ID=6430. Accessed February 5, 2020.
11. Gilk T. RSNA Scientific Presentation, "MRI Accidents and Adverse Events". 2012. Available at: https://www.youtube.com/watch?v=c-iMRYXhIzg. Accessed February 5, 2020.
12. Delfino JG, Krainak DM, Flesher SA, et al. MRI-related FDA adverse event reports: A 10-yr review. Med Phys 2019;46:5562–71. Available at: https://aapm.onlinelibrary.wiley.com/doi/10.1002/mp.13768. Accessed August 25, 2020.
13. "Reducing MRI accidents" infographic. Metrasens. 2019. Available at: https://www.metrasens.com/mri-safety/mri-safety-infographic/. Accessed February 5, 2020.
14. Guidelines for design and construction of health care facilities. St Louis (MO): Facilities Guideline Institute; 2014. Available at: https://fgiguidelines.org/guidelines/2014-fgi-guidelines/. Accessed April 19, 2020.
15. Guidelines for design and construction of health care facilities. St Louis (MO): Facilities Guideline Institute; 2018. Available at: https://fgiguidelines.org/guidelines/2018-fgi-guidelines/. Accessed April 19, 2020.
16. Gosbee J, Gosbee LL. "Flying object hits MRI", PSnet. Available at: https://psnet.ahrq.gov/web-mm/flying-object-hits-mri. Accessed February 5, 2020.
17. Gilk T. "Designing and engineering MRI safety", American Society of Healthcare Engineering. 2008. Available at: https://www.ashe.org/mri. Accessed February 5, 2020.

Elements of Effective Patient Screening to Improve Safety in MRI

Vera Kimbrell, BSRT, R MR FSMRT[a,b,*]

KEYWORDS

- MR Safety • Screening • MR Safe • MR Conditional • MR Unsafe • MRI Safety • Ferrous
- Nonferrous

KEY POINTS

- Rationale for screening—to adequately protect the magnetic resonance (MR) environment, including patients, staff, and equipment, a barrier to access must be in place. Each individual and patient who enters Zone 3 and Zone 4 must pass a medical and physical screening process.
- Access control—only those individuals or equipment that have been screened are allowed in the MR environment (Zone 3 and Zone 4). A Level 2 MR staff member determines access after careful review of medical history and removal of metallic objects.
- Training for Level 1 and Level 2 staff—MR personnel working in the environment must be trained and understand all safety concerns. These individuals are responsible for all individuals and equipment entering the scan room (Zone 4).
- Screening process—each facility or clinic must develop an internal system to prescreen, review the day of the examination, and perform a final stop to double-check for metal internal or external to the patient just prior to entry to the examination room (Zone 4).
- MR conditional and safe equipment—screening also be must done on any equipment used or brought into the MR examination room. After careful review and investigation, this equipment must be labeled either safe or conditional for use in Zone 4.

TERMINOLOGY

Ferrous

Ferrous refers to a material that has a significant amount of iron and has an attractive interaction with the magnetic resonance (MR) scanner.

Nonferrous

Nonferrous refers to material that has no iron components and no attractive force a magnetic force.

Zones 1 to 4

The Zones 1 to 4 safety areas are designated in an MR facility in order to prevent unscreened individuals from entering potentially unsafe areas.

Zone 1—safe for the general public. No screening required, everyone could enter this area.

Zone 2—no screening is required, but this area is for designated hospital personnel and often includes MR patient preparation area. Zone 2 typically is the designated code area for emergent procedures and may require signage to restrict the general public.

Zone 3—this area is for Level 1 and Level 2 trained personnel, screened staff, and patients or research subjects who have undergone screening, been cleared for Zone 4, are changed into MR appropriate attire, and removed all external metal objects and devices.

[a] Brigham and Women's Hospital, Boston, MA, USA; [b] SMRT Safety Committee 2020, 66 Bellingham Street, Mendon, MA 01756, USA
* 66 Bellingham Street, Mendon, MA 01756.
E-mail address: bvdmiller@mac.com

Magn Reson Imaging Clin N Am 28 (2020) 489–496
https://doi.org/10.1016/j.mric.2020.07.005
1064-9689/20/© 2020 Elsevier Inc. All rights reserved.

Zone 4—the scan room itself, which houses the MR magnet. This area has constantly active magnetic fields and requires that all individuals and equipment be cleared prior to entry.

Level 1 Trained Personnel

Level 1 trained personnel are individuals who have received formal education in general MR safety concepts, have completed instruction in screening procedures, and are able to function safely in the MR environment. Yearly refresher training and testing are required, and screening of those staff should be done at least annually. These staff members are reminded to self-report any change in medical history that might have an impact on their MR access and must follow all MR safety and hospital policies.

Level 2 Trained Personnel

Level 2 MR training includes an advanced knowledge of MR safety. This level usually is designated for MR technologists, radiographers, and radiologists (MDs or equivalent) who are educated to make decisions about MR safety and access for patients and staff. They can review and approve equipment, implants, and individuals to enter Zone 4.

Magnetic Resonance Safe

MR safe refers to an object or device that poses no threat to safety and can be used freely in the MR environment. The object or device does not contain any metal and cannot act as a conductor.

Magnetic Resonance Conditional

MR conditional refers to an object or device that has specific conditions for safe use and is not completely safe inherently. This object or device may be used in the MR environment, assuming the conditions for safe use are strictly met.

Magnetic Resonance Unsafe

MR unsafe refers to an object or device that poses a safety threat on or in a patient or research subject in the MR environment. There are no conditions that can make the object or device conditionally safe in the MR environment.

ELEMENTS OF EFFECTIVE PATIENT SCREENING TO IMPROVE SAFETY IN MAGNETIC RESONANCE RATIONALE

MRI examinations involve strong magnetic and radiofrequency (RF) electromagnetic fields, both of which have inherent safety concerns for staff, patients, and equipment. The rapidly evolving science of MRI involves dangers not well understood by those who benefit from its technology. This modality is an extremely valuable diagnostic tool and important to clinical and research practices. For a majority of examinations, MRI is a safe and noninvasive procedure. There are underlying safety concerns, however, that, if not addressed and alleviated, can cause harm and even death.[3–5] Anyone who enters the MR environment both be should screened for the examination and have at least rudimentary knowledge to function safely in the scan room. To accomplish this task, MR professionals employ a mixture of signage, safety training, access control, and screening for those entering Zone 3 and Zone 4.[1,2,4]

Numerous groups and organizations have outlined the basics of MR screening in published guidelines and white papers.[1,2,5,6] These guideline documents are well researched and tested. They are designed to protect patients, research subjects, and those who work in the environment. In addition to MR personnel and patients, nursing, anesthesia, maintenance, and other hospital workers may require periodic entry to the MR environment. To mitigate risk and provide a safe and uneventful examination experience, the MR professional staff must perform a thorough screening and risk assessment for each person who enters the MR environment. MR professionals spend an increasingly significant amount of their workday researching, reviewing, and evaluating implant data to ensure the safety of all persons requiring access or diagnostic imaging. The process of by which this is accomplished must be an ingrained part of an institution's safety plan and daily workflow.[5]

The practice of communicating safety risks to the staff and radiologists and screening individuals prior to admission to Zone 4 should be documented via an MR site's policy and procedures. Addressed in the policy should be requirements for access control and training of any person(s) traversing Zone 3 and Zone 4.[1,4–6] These policies should be easily accessible and followed to the letter each and every interaction. Policies should be reviewed and updated at least annually to ensure they are current and encompass any new workflow or updates to procedures.

Responsibility for MR safety is the purview of the MR medical director (MRMD) and ultimately the health care institution. Level 1 and Level 2 personnel typically handle the majority of day-to-day interactions. At many institutions, there are an MR safety officer (MRSO) and an MR safety expert (MRSE); their roles along with the MRMD's make up the backbone of the safety program and the MR safety committee.[7] The MR safety committee is tasked with maintaining a safe physical environment, up-to-date policy and procedures, consistent training, and restricted access control for Zone 3 and Zone 4.

RISKS

Due the strong magnetic and RF electromagnetic fields that are necessary for MR imaging, inherent risks involved must be understood. Projectiles from ferrous metal and induced currents leading to potential burns can cause serious consequences and even death.[3,7] MR professionals must know and understand the principles of magnetism and electromagnetic fields in order to create and maintain a safe environment. The dangers of exposure to the static magnetic field (B_0) and RF electromagnetic fields (B_1) are not widely known or completely understood by typical patients, research subjects, or those who require only occasional access to the MRI environment. Therefore, effective screening procedures are necessary to prevent unsafe exposures. MR professionals are tasked with the responsibility of identifying any potential safety risk and ensuring safety for all involved.

PHYSICAL LAYOUT AND WORKFLOW

Among the most underappreciated aspects of MR safety are the design of the site and ability of the staff to manage workflow. When a new site is planned, consideration for how the staff will manage patient flow within the 4 prescribed safety zones can have an enormous impact on both efficiency and sustainability of MR safety practices. Consulting with the safety committee along with the site managers and staff technologists/radiographers prior to construction may alleviate the need for costly refits or necessitating staff to find workarounds for maintaining safe practices. An example of this is sites with small footprints, whose safety zones do not allow for restricted access. Planning for critically ill patients and life-supporting equipment may involve extra space for transfer, waveguides for lines and wires, and designated areas in the examination room for MR conditional equipment. For sites that may have preexisting construction and are attempting to conform to existing space, careful attention should be paid to the ability to interview, screen, and change patients prior to entering restricted areas. Site access control is imperative to MR safety practices.[1,4]

SCREENING PROCEDURE FOR PATIENTS AND RESEARCH SUBJECTS

As part of safety screening workflow in MRI, the environment is laid out into safety zones. There typically are 4 areas with increasing need for intervention. Zone 1 and Zone 2 do not require screening of individuals, but Zone 3 and Zone 4 necessitate written and verbal safety checks before entry. All existing metal, either internal or external, must be identified, removed, or investigated for MR safety prior to proceeding into the MR environment. This step is critical to keeping both the individual and staff safe and must be part of all safety workflows. Only those who have completed MR Level 1 and/or Level 2 training are allowed to move freely in these areas or make decisions about patient or equipment suitability to enter Zone 3 or Zone 4.[1,4] Sites must ensure the physical layout incorporates methods to keep the general public and ancillary hospital staff from inadvertently moving into an area that would cause harm. Although this may create issues for delivery of goods, cleaning, and workflow, it is essential to the success of a safety program.

Per American College of Radiology (ACR) requirements,[1,2,5] most sites use either badge swipe access or keypads to secure the entry to Zone 3 and Zone 4 areas. It is extremely important that the doors to both Zone 3 and Zone 4 are closed at all times and accessed only when patients or staff requires entry. Inability to secure the entry points when trained personnel are not present can lead to serious incidents[3] (**Fig. 1**).

PREPROCEDURE SCREENING

The accepted screening process in most institutions involves 3 steps. The initial phase requires

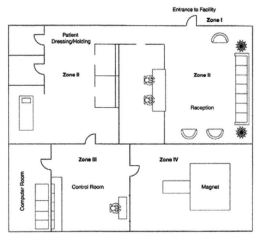

Fig. 1. ACR safety zones. (*From* ACR safety zones https://www.acr.org/Clinical-Resources/Radiology-Safety/MR-Safety; with permission.)

a questionnaire carried out remotely via phone confirmation or perhaps an e-mailed computer survey. The use of patient portals with access to the MRI screening form is another option for patients who want to complete the MRI safety screening form in the electronic health record. This typically involves a series of questions designed to elicit pertinent medical history as well as instructions to arrive at the institution prepared to change into MR safe hospital attire. Instructions also should be provided to the patients about cosmetics and body piercings prior to their MR examination. If any red flags are raised during this phase, the MR team can begin research and identification of potential safety issues. Having a comprehensive screening prior to the patients' arrival has proved critical to an efficient workflow, because it can take a great deal of time and effort to investigate surgical history and identify devices. Many devices require intervention, additional staff, or in some cases the patient might not be able to be scanned at a particular facility or individual MR scanner. Dealing with these issues at the time of scan can lead to frustration and potential rescheduling of the examination.[6,8] All efforts made to prescreen and instruct patients prior to the scan date facilitate workflow and contribute to a positive safety culture (**Fig. 2**).

RESEARCHING AND CLEARING OF IMPLANTS AND DEVICES

When the medical history review yields an implanted internal or external on-planted biomedical device, careful review must transpire. The precise make and model of the device must be identified carefully so that Level 2 staff members can assess the device as safe, conditional, or unsafe relative to the MR environment. This is accomplished through examination of the electronic medical record, verbal communication with the patient or family, and manufacturer support and safety information, along with site policy and procedures. Most manufacturers of devices have performed MR safety testing and can provide this information if requested. Typically, safety information is available on the Web site for the implant vendor or by organizations who perform independent testing. Level 2 staff compile this information to determine scanning capabilities. MR safe devices do not need intervention and may be imaged readily. MR conditional devices require a greater level of scrutiny. Some devices are easily cleared and scanned following easily achievable conditional guidelines, but others may be more complex and the conditions not easily met. In these cases, the supervising radiologist must make the final decision, potentially with

A

MAGNETIC RESONANCE (MR) PROCEDURE SCREENING FORM FOR PATIENTS

Date ____/____/____ Patient Number ____________

Name ______________________ (Last name, First name, Middle Initial) Age ______ Height ______ Weight ______

Date of Birth ____/____/____ (month, day, year) Male ☐ Female ☐ Body Part to be Examined ____________

Address ______________________ Telephone (home) (____) ____-______

City ______________________ Telephone (work) (____) ____-______

State ____________ Zip Code ________

Reason for MRI and/or Symptoms ______________________

Referring Physician ______________________ Telephone (____) ____-______

1. Have you had prior surgery or an operation (e.g., arthroscopy, endoscopy, etc.) of any kind? ☐ No ☐ Yes
   If yes, please indicate the date and type of surgery:
   Date ____/____/____ Type of surgery ____________
   Date ____/____/____ Type of surgery ____________
2. Have you had a prior diagnostic imaging study or examination (MRI, CT, Ultrasound, X-ray, etc.)? ☐ No ☐ Yes
   If yes, please list: Body part / Date / Facility
   MRI ______ ____/____/____ ______
   CT/CAT Scan ______ ____/____/____ ______
   X-Ray ______ ____/____/____ ______
   Ultrasound ______ ____/____/____ ______
   Nuclear Medicine ______ ____/____/____ ______
   Other______ ______ ____/____/____ ______
3. Have you experienced any problem related to a previous MRI examination or MR procedure? ☐ No ☐ Yes
   If yes, please describe: ____________
4. Have you had an injury to the eye involving a metallic object or fragment (e.g., metallic slivers, shavings, foreign body, etc.)? ☐ No ☐ Yes
   If yes, please describe: ____________
5. Have you ever been injured by a metallic object or foreign body (e.g., BB, bullet, shrapnel, etc.)? ☐ No ☐ Yes
   If yes, please describe: ____________
6. Are you currently taking or have you recently taken any medication or drug? ☐ No ☐ Yes
   If yes, please list: ____________
7. Are you allergic to any medication? ☐ No ☐ Yes
   If yes, please list: ____________
8. Do you have a history of asthma, allergic reaction, respiratory disease, or reaction to a contrast medium or dye used for an MRI, CT, or X-ray examination? ☐ No ☐ Yes
9. Do you have anemia or any disease(s) that affects your blood, a history of renal (kidney) disease, renal (kidney) failure, renal (kidney) transplant, high blood pressure (hypertension), liver (hepatic) disease, a history of diabetes, or seizures? ☐ No ☐ Yes
   If yes, please describe: ____________

For female patients:

10. Date of last menstrual period: ____/____/____ Post menopausal? ☐ No ☐ Yes
11. Are you pregnant or experiencing a late menstrual period? ☐ No ☐ Yes
12. Are you taking oral contraceptives or receiving hormonal treatment? ☐ No ☐ Yes
13. Are you taking any type of fertility medication or having fertility treatments? ☐ No ☐ Yes
    If yes, please describe: ____________
14. Are you currently breastfeeding? ☐ No ☐ Yes

B

WARNING: Certain implants, devices, or objects may be hazardous to you and/or may interfere with the MR procedure (i.e., MRI, MR angiography, functional MRI, MR spectroscopy). Do not enter the MR system room or MR environment if you have any question or concern regarding an implant, device, or object. Consult the MRI Technologist or Radiologist BEFORE entering the MR system room. The MR system magnet is ALWAYS on.

Please indicate if you have any of the following:

- ☐ Yes ☐ No Aneurysm clip(s)
- ☐ Yes ☐ No Cardiac pacemaker
- ☐ Yes ☐ No Implanted cardioverter defibrillator (ICD)
- ☐ Yes ☐ No Electronic implant or device
- ☐ Yes ☐ No Magnetically-activated implant or device
- ☐ Yes ☐ No Neurostimulation system
- ☐ Yes ☐ No Spinal cord stimulator
- ☐ Yes ☐ No Internal electrodes or wires
- ☐ Yes ☐ No Bone growth/bone fusion stimulator
- ☐ Yes ☐ No Cochlear, otologic, or other ear implant
- ☐ Yes ☐ No Insulin or other infusion pump
- ☐ Yes ☐ No Implanted drug infusion device
- ☐ Yes ☐ No Any type of prosthesis (eye, penile, etc.)
- ☐ Yes ☐ No Heart valve prosthesis
- ☐ Yes ☐ No Eyelid spring or wire
- ☐ Yes ☐ No Artificial or prosthetic limb
- ☐ Yes ☐ No Metallic stent, filter, or coil
- ☐ Yes ☐ No Shunt (spinal or intraventricular)
- ☐ Yes ☐ No Vascular access port and/or catheter
- ☐ Yes ☐ No Radiation seeds or implants
- ☐ Yes ☐ No Swan-Ganz or thermodilution catheter
- ☐ Yes ☐ No Medication patch (Nicotine, Nitroglycerine)
- ☐ Yes ☐ No Any metallic fragment or foreign body
- ☐ Yes ☐ No Wire mesh implant
- ☐ Yes ☐ No Tissue expander (e.g., breast)
- ☐ Yes ☐ No Surgical staples, clips, or metallic sutures
- ☐ Yes ☐ No Joint replacement (hip, knee, etc.)
- ☐ Yes ☐ No Bone/joint pin, screw, nail, wire, plate, etc.
- ☐ Yes ☐ No IUD, diaphragm, or pessary
- ☐ Yes ☐ No Are you here for an MRI examination?
- ☐ Yes ☐ No Dentures or partial plates
- ☐ Yes ☐ No Tattoo or permanent makeup
- ☐ Yes ☐ No Body piercing jewelry
- ☐ Yes ☐ No Hearing aid *(Remove before entering MR system room)*
- ☐ Yes ☐ No Other implant ____________
- ☐ Yes ☐ No Breathing problem or motion disorder

Please mark on the figure(s) below the location of any implant or metal inside of or on your body.

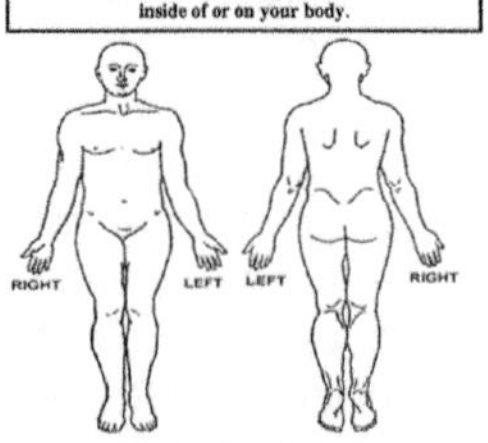

IMPORTANT INSTRUCTIONS

Before entering the MR environment or MR system room, you must remove all metallic objects including hearing aids, dentures, partial plates, keys, beeper, cell phone, eyeglasses, hair pins, barrettes, jewelry, body piercing jewelry, watch, safety pins, paperclips, money clip, credit cards, bank cards, magnetic strip cards, coins, pens, pocket knife, nail clipper, tools, clothing with metal fasteners, & clothing with metallic threads.

Please consult the MRI Technologist or Radiologist if you have any question or concern BEFORE you enter the MR system room.

NOTE: You may be advised or required to wear earplugs or other hearing protection during the MR procedure to prevent possible problems or hazards related to acoustic noise.

I attest that the above information is correct to the best of my knowledge. I read and understand the contents of this form and had the opportunity to ask questions regarding the information on this form and regarding the MR procedure that I am about to undergo.

Signature of Person Completing Form: ____________ (Signature) Date ____/____/____

Form Completed By: ☐ Patient ☐ Relative ☐ Nurse ____________ (Print name) ____________ (Relationship to patient)

Form Information Reviewed By: ____________ (Print name) ____________ (Signature)

☐ MRI Technologist ☐ Nurse ☐ Radiologist ☐ Other____________

Fig. 2. MR screening form. (*Courtesy of* Dr. Frank Shellock at mrisafety.com; with permission.)

consultation with a designated MRSE, carefully weighing risk versus benefit for the individual case. [1,4,8] For any unsafe or unknown implants, a significant approval process is needed with a risk-benefit assessment approved by the site's MRMD.

DAY OF THE EXAMINATION SCREENING

Once a patient arrives at the MR facility, Level 2 trained MR personnel review previously obtained screening information, perform a secondary check, and interview the patient for all items on the screening form, ensuring the proper identification of any implants. This ensures the patient or subject understands the form and has an opportunity to ask any questions they might have about the examination and safety issues. After the patient is thoroughly screened, the next step is to escort them to a dressing area where the patient changes out of their personal clothing and into hospital/clinic attire. Most sites have a combination of gowns, robes, pants, and footwear to ensure patients are comfortable and modestly dressed. This step is extremely important because RF electromagnetic fields can induce a current that may lead to heating and the potential for RF burns. Metal and metallic fibers in the area of transmitted RF are a significant safety concern. There have been reports of serious incidents with athletic t-shirts, underwear and other metallic solution (antimicrobial)–infused clothing.[9] Allowing patients to retain personal clothing for their MR examination is not considered a safe practice and should not be allowed. Here is an example of inappropriate clothing for an MR examination: https://www.yathletics.com/products/long-sleeve-crew.

Patients may be hesitant to remove their personal apparel. To alleviate this concern, alerting them during the initial screening call is recommended. Policies should be in place to respectfully address patient clothing required due to religious constraints. Signage in the dressing rooms and reminders by the technologist prior to changing can aid nervous or anxious patients. A simple reminder of the need to be safe in the MR environment might smooth over complaints. The ability to communicate with and elicit accurate information about internal and external metal or devices is imperative to MR screening and safety during the procedure. Language barriers and physical limitations may be obstacles to effective screening and compliance with MR appropriate clothing. Whenever possible, extra time, interpreter services, or help from family members should be incorporated into the patient preparation. Support provided by family members in Zone 3 and Zone 4 require appropriate screening and metal removal. These difficulties can sometimes be anticipated during the prescreening process and prior accommodations make for the examination date.[5]

For those patients who may not be ambulatory and arrive by wheelchair or stretcher, an additional transfer to MR conditional or MR safe equipment may be needed. An assessment of all bedding, ancillary equipment, and the person's clothing must be performed. Leads, patches, and other unsafe objects must be discovered and investigated prior to crossing into Zone 4. This process can be difficult with patients who are extremely ill and traveling with life-supporting equipment. Prior communication with nursing staff can help to address concerns in advance, communicate the screening process, and alleviate unnecessary steps during the transfer process. Here is an example of appropriate MR attire: https://www.walmart.com/ip/Hospital-Gowns.

SCREENING IMMEDIATELY PRIOR TO ZONE 4

The third and final step in the screening process transpires at the door to Zone 4, where the scan takes place. At this time, the patient should have completed verbal and either written or electronic screening as well as be attired in MRI-appropriate dress. As a final safety pause, however, the MR Level 2 trained technologist makes a last check of screening questions just prior to crossing the threshold. Although this step might seem excessive, many forgotten items or information have been reported anecdotally during this process. Presence of a written time-out checklist, especially for patients who cannot communicate, should be documented for each examination.[5,6,8]

A recent ACR guidance document on MR safety recommended the use of the final stop or time-out process in the most recent 2019 update.[6] Following this best practice guideline allows MR personnel to make a final review with patients, staff, and equipment to ensure all safety procedures are in place and all metal has been removed or evaluated.[6,8]

Some sites have incorporated the use of ferrous metal detectors (FMDs) in the changing area and/or at the door of the examination room (Zone 4). These tools can be used as adjuncts to the screening process and provide an additional layer of security when screening for ferrous objects.[10] The FMDs are designed to produce visual and/or auditory alarms if ferrous metal is detected. When used to augment patient screening in Zone 2, an FMD system has been shown effective in identifying the presence of implanted pacemakers and defibrillators.[11] Although they may not provide remediation for nonferrous metal or the potential for heating or burns, they can prevent catastrophic accidents when ferrous metal inadvertently is introduced to Zone 4. Several types of FMDs exist for use in the MR environment. It is recommended that the site carefully evaluate the physical layout as well as workflow prior to purchasing, installing, and implementing these tools. Improper use can lead to alarm fatigue and decrease the effectiveness of this adjunct screening process.[12] FMDs are an adjunct to MR safety and screening but should not replace other written, verbal, or physical screening processes (**Fig. 3**).

NONPATIENT/SUBJECT SCREENING

There are many divergent types of individuals who may need access to Zone 4 to perform a variety of duties. Researchers, medical personnel, maintenance, and visitors may have a legitimate need to enter the MR scanning area. These individuals are not imaged and, therefore, not susceptible to the RF magnetic fields. The static main magnetic field, however, is a safety risk to all and the same screening scrutiny must apply to the casual visitor. Unfettered access to Zone 4 must be tightly managed and given only to those who have been trained, screened, and deemed acceptable to

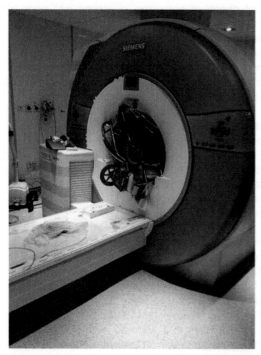

Fig. 3. Ferrous wheelchair attracted to MR scanner. (*Courtesy of* KOPP Development, Inc., Barcelona, Spain; with permission.)

function in the environment. Depending on the level of access, amount of time that will be spent, or the circumstances of the request, differing levels of screening and training may be involved. These requests should be triaged and a policy to provide necessary screening, training, and access developed. A secondary screening form designed specifically for these individuals who are not being scanned should be made available.

SHORT-TERM OR EPISODIC SCREENING

In order to be granted access to an MRI environment where a strong magnetic field exists, an individual must undergo a vigorous screening even for a single trip into Zone 4. An example of this is a parent who wishes to accompany their child or the friend or spouse of an anxious patient. To the general population, screening may seem excessive for a brief period of exposure, but MR personnel must never let down their guard and are entrusted with the safety of all whom need to enter the scan room (Zone 4). Prior to allowing entry, the individual should be screened in print or electronically depending on the system. All ferrous objects must be removed; internal devices identified, and the individual cleared by a Level 2 trained MR staff member. If the individual needs future admission, the paper or electronic screening information should be retained in the site's employee records and updated if changes occur. The screening procedure and removal of all ferrous metal must be done each time for every person entering Zone 4.

LONG-TERM ACCESS FOR STAFF

For those individuals who work daily in the MR environment, more intensive training and responsibility for safety is expected. These individuals typically are MR technologists, radiographers, nurses, and physicians who handle MR procedures and the safety of all patients and hospital staff on a daily basis. Those staff members should have at least Level 1 training, and, for those making decisions about entry to the MR scanner (Zone 4), Level 2 training is mandatory. All persons and equipment that cross the barrier to Zone 4 should be examined and approved by an individual with Level 2 safety training.[6,8] This review entails an advanced understanding of the risks involved in MR procedures and the ability to mitigate those risks to a safe level. Managing busy acute care sites can be challenging, because patients may require intervention from multiple hospital staff members. Although it is tempting to forego the usual screening and approval steps, it is important to remember that most significant MR accidents happened during stressful situations when a person's guard is let down.[3]

ALTERNATIVE SCREENING METHODS

There are many instances where conventional screening methods are not possible. Patients may have language barriers or difficulty communicating or may not be alert and oriented. These patients could require interpreter services, help from family members or even at times radiologic imaging to investigate the potential for implants or devices. For each distinct case, a risk-benefit assessment clearance by the supervising radiologist is required to evaluate the need for an MR examination. The benefits are weighed against the potential risks from unknown implants or metallic fragments. Along with a physical examination of the patient for external devices and scars that may indicate the presence of an implanted device, radiographs and CT examinations may provide clearance or the need for further investigation. Ferromagnetic detectors may be able to add valuable information. Medical records, if available, may help MR personnel research and understand a patient's medical and surgical history. These situations can be complex and take both time and resources; however, screening must be completed prior to every patient's entry into Zone 4 and the magnet itself.

EQUIPMENT AND SUPPLIES

The use of supplies, transport equipment, and medical assist devices is a necessary component of any hospital environment. Careful consideration is given to the purchase of wheelchairs, stretchers, intravenous poles, and all other equipment needed to perform patient care in the MR environment. Level 2 safety personnel must review all information relative to a given device prior to exposure to Zone 4 (scan room). Many companies now are producing MR safe and MR conditional devices for use in during the MR procedures. Careful review of the manufacturer guidelines assists the MR staff in the safe and effective use of equipment in the MR environment.

Either a strong handheld test magnet or FMD can help make determinations about safety relative to translational and attractive forces from the magnet field. Induced currents from RF leading to burns can be prevented by careful prevention of any skin-to-skin contact and/or the presence of loops, metal, or wires. Level 2 MR personnel must be present to assess interactions with monitoring equipment or other life-saving devices. Level 2 MR staff are trained to understand proper positioning of the

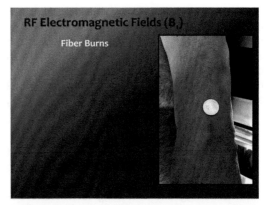

Fig. 4. MR-related thermal burn. (*Courtesy of* Anne Marie Sawyer, BS, RT(R)(MR), FSMRT, Charleston, SC.)

patient, proper placement of insulating pads between the patient and bore wall, and necessary equipment prior to the commencement of the imaging session. A careful appraisal of equipment in use during the examination must be conducted and MR conditions met prior to commencement of the MR examination. Failure to properly perform this level of screening and assessment has led to significant harm[1,4–6] (**Fig. 4**).

SUMMARY

Screening is the primary process by which MR professionals safeguard against ferrous metal projectile accidents and RF burns. The primary elements of effective screening workflow incorporate prescreening, ideally several days prior to the appointment, day of examination review, and at-the-door checks prior to any person or equipment's entry to Zone 4. All members of the MR team should have Level 1 MR training, and anyone making access decisions should maintain Level 2 MR safety training. It is recommended that training be repeated yearly to help staff remain current in all MR safety procedures.[6] Researching implanted devices and patient-related equipment is the purview of a Level 2 trained staff member,[7,8] some of whom may be MRSOs. This individual must sign off for entry into Zone 4 by anyone or anything. Regardless of the need to commence work and maintain throughput, screening always must take place. Using consistent and repetitive questioning, Level 1 and Level 2 team members extract information relative to surgical history, external objects, and the potential for hidden or unreported metallic devices. Questioning alone cannot solve all issues. MR staff reviews appropriate available medical history, questions family members, and employs FMDs when available. A combination of these processes and tools is considered best practice when preparing patients, research subjects, or staff to enter Zone 4. Along with access restriction, safety training, effective policies and procedures, and support from the MR safety committee, MR staff can maintain safety for everyone in the MR environment. There are no exceptions to the pursuit of MR safety and the care of patients and staff members.

CLINICS CARE POINTS

- MRI is an excellent diagnostic tool for most patients when appropriate safety precautions are taken.
- Interviewing and screening for metallic objects, electronic devices, and copper-infused fabrics can prevent most MRI accidents.
- Training of all personnel in MR safety and appropriate patient preparation ensures a better workflow and an overall safer MRI environment.
- With proper explanation and attention to individual comfort, most patients can understand and adhere to safety policies and procedures.
- All persons and equipment that enter the MRI-restricted areas (Zones 3 and 4) must be screened and deemed safe or conditional prior to entry.
- Accidents can be prevented with education, screening, and training in MRI safety principles.

DISCLOSURE

The author has no financial disclosures in relation to MR safety or the content of this publication.

REFERENCES

1. "MR safety guidance, documents and links." ISMRM; 2019. Available at: https://www.ismrm.org/mr-safety-links/mr-safety-resources-page/.
2. ACR. "MR Safety." American College of Radiology. Available at: https://www.acr.org/Clinical-Resources/Radiology-Safety/MR-Safety http://mriquestions.com/acr-safety-zones.html. "ACR Safety Zones." Questions and Answers in MRI.
3. Peck P. "Fatal MRI accident is first of its kind." WebMD, WebMD 2001. Available at: https://www.webmd.com/a-to-z-guides/news/20010801/fatal-mri-accident-is-first-of-its-kind#1.
4. Henderson JM, Tkach J, Phillips M, et al. Permanent neurological deficit related to magnetic resonance imaging in a patient with implanted deep brain stimulation electrodes for parkinson's disease: case report. Neurosurgery 2005;57(5):E1063. Available at: www.ncbi.nlm.nih.gov/pubmed/16284543.
5. Greenberg TD, Tkach J, Phillips M, et al. ACR guidance document on MR safe practices: updates and critical information 2019." Wiley Online Library, John Wiley & Sons, Ltd; 2019. Available at:https://onlinelibrary.wiley.com/doi/full/10.1002/jmri.26880.
6. Sawyer-Glover AM, Shellock FG. "Pre-MRI procedure screening: recommendations and safety considerations for biomedical implants and devices." J Magn Reson Imaging 2000;12(1):92–106.
7. Calamante F, et al. Recommended responsibilities for management of MR safety." Wiley Online Library, John Wiley & Sons, Ltd; 2016. Available at:www.onlinelibrary.wiley.com/doi/full/10.1002/jmri.25282.
8. Shellock FG, Alberto S. "MRI Safety Update 2008: Part 2, Screening Patients for MRI." Am J Roentgenol 2008;191(4):1140–9.
9. Pietryga JA, Fonder MA, Rogg JM, et al. Invisible metallic microfiber in clothing presents unrecognized MRI risk for cutaneous burn. AJNR Am J Neuroradiol 2013;34(5):E47–50. Available at: http://www.ajnr.org/content/34/5/E47.
10. "Using the 2018 guidelines from the joint commission to kickstart your hospital's program to reduce opioid-induced ventilatory impairment." Anesthesia Patient Safety Foundation. Available at: https://www.apsf.org/article/using-the-2018-guidelines-from-the-joint-commission-to-kickstart-your-hospitals-program-to-reduce-opioid-induced-ventilatory-impairment/.
11. Watson RE, Walsh SM, Felmlee JP, et al. Augmenting MRI safety screening processes: reliable identification of cardiac implantable electronic devices by a ferromagnetic detector system. J Magn Reson Imaging 2019;49(7):e297–9.
12. Orchard LJ. "Implementation of a Ferromagnetic Detection System in a Clinical MRI Setting." Radiography 2015;21(3):248–53. Available at: www.sciencedirect.com/science/article/pii/S1078817414001606.

MR Imaging Safety Considerations of Gadolinium-Based Contrast Agents
Gadolinium Retention and Nephrogenic Systemic Fibrosis

Jennifer S. McDonald, PhD*, Robert J. McDonald, MD, PhD

KEYWORDS

• Gadolinium-based contrast agents • Gadolinium retention • Nephrogenic systemic fibrosis
• MR imaging contrast agent • Radiology safety • Gadolinium deposition disease

KEY POINTS

• Gadolinium (Gd) is retained in tissues and organs, including brain, of patients after intravenous exposure to Gd-based contrast agents (GBCAs).
• Higher amounts of Gd retention are observed with linear versus macrocyclic GBCAs, although there is variability within GBCA classes.
• The clinical relevance of Gd retention, if any, currently is not known.

INTRODUCTION

Gadolinium (Gd)-based contrast agents (GBCAs) have greatly expanded the clinical utility of MR imaging in identification of diseases that otherwise would be undetectable with unenhanced MR imaging or other imaging modalities.[1,2] Consequently, more than 450 million GBCA doses have been administered worldwide since initial regulatory approval in 1988.[3,4] The historic safety profile of GBCAs has been highly favorable, with very low rates of adverse side effects compared with other pharmaceuticals, including iodinated contrast agents.[2–4]

Because free Gd is cytotoxic, the in vivo safety of GBCAs is conferred via its chelated form; the organic ligand serves as a physiologic chaperone, allowing this toxic rare earth metal to be safely administered intravenously and excreted, primarily via renal clearance.[1] At the time of initial regulatory approval, it was widely thought that the Gd ion remained in the chelated state after intravenous administration of GBCAs and was excreted rapidly in the urine as an intact chelate. A rapidly growing body of literature has emerged, however, to refute this belief, with convincing evidence of dose-dependent Gd accumulation in many if not all tissues of patients exposed to a GBCA, even in the setting of normal renal function.[5,6] Although tissue retention appears to be highest with linear GBCAs, all agents demonstrate some degree of tissue retention of Gd in some form.[7–10]

These recent findings have prompted new concerns from patients, clinicians, and regulatory authorities. In response to these concerns and data showing higher Gd retention after linear GBCA exposure compared with macrocyclic GBCA use, the European Medicines Agency largely has suspended clinical use of linear GBCAs.[11] In contrast, the US Food and Drug Administration (FDA)

Department of Radiology, Mayo Clinic, 200 1st Street Southwest, Rochester, MN 55905, USA
* Corresponding author.
E-mail address: mcdonald.jennifer@mayo.edu

Magn Reson Imaging Clin N Am 28 (2020) 497–507
https://doi.org/10.1016/j.mric.2020.06.001
1064-9689/20/© 2020 Elsevier Inc. All rights reserved.

concluded that no regulatory product suspension(s) were warranted as of 2019, although further investigation into the safety of these agents is needed and ongoing.[12] Such differences in regulatory actions reflect differences in regulatory risk tolerance and risk mitigation policies and underscore the need for additional investigation into the safety of these agents.[11–13]

CHEMICAL PROPERTIES AND STABILITIES OF GADOLINIUM-BASED CONTRAST AGENTS

Since 1988, 9 distinct GBCA chelates with unique chemical and physical properties have been developed; as of 2020, 6 of these agents remain in active clinical use in the United States (**Table 1**).[3] GBCAs can be classified by the identity of the organic polyaminocarboxylate ligand (linear vs macrocyclic agent classes), charge (ionic vs nonionic), protein binding and associated relaxivity effects, thermodynamic stability, and kinetic lability. Central to the current concern is the relative instability and kinetic lability of GBCA chelates, which are consequences of the need for a labile H_2O:Gd bond, required for effective bulk water proton relaxation.[14] In general, macrocyclic GBCAs are more kinetically inert (less likely to dissociate over a period of time) than linear GBCAs, despite, in some cases, similar or inferior thermodynamic stabilities of macrocyclic compared with linear GBCAs.

Accordingly, all GBCAs theoretically exist in a complex chemical equilibrium with dechelated free Gd, free ligand, and myriad endogenous inorganic and biological chelates, governed by their unique thermodynamic (affinity of the ligand for the Gd ion at equilibrium) and kinetic stabilities (rate of approach to equilibrium). Dechelated forms of Gd in vivo are numerous and include free forms that associate with anionic counterions (eg, Cl^- and PO_4^{3-}), forms that associate with negatively charged biopolymers (eg, protein side chains and nucleic acid phosphate diester backbones), and insoluble precipitates.[15] In addition to these dechelated forms, Gd also may be retained long term as an intact GBCA chelate.[16,17]

BIODISTRIBUTION

The short-term biodistribution and pharmacokinetics of intravenously administered GBCAs have been studied extensively in preclinical models and humans. Almost all (>90%) intravenously administered GBCAs are cleared via the kidneys within 24 hours, with slower clearance in patients with renal insufficiency.[18] Long-term clearance of GBCAs and Gd is less well understood, with few studies examining clearance of GBCAs more than 24 hours after exposure. In these limited studies, many patients had detectable levels of Gd in their urine weeks to years after GBCA exposure. These findings suggest a complex biodistribution multicompartment model with 1 or more deep compartments from which chronically retained Gd is slowly released,[19–21] such as bone, liver, and other organs. In both animals and humans, bone appears to be a major reservoir for Gd in vivo, where Gd is actively incorporated into bone matrix as Ca-replaced hydroxyapatite by osteoblasts.[16] In 1 study, bone retention was detected in patients up to 8 years after injection.[16] Animal studies have shown detectable levels of Gd in tissues at intermediate (1–2 weeks after injection) and long-term (34–52 weeks after injection) time points.[22–25] In these studies, higher concentrations of Gd typically were observed with linear versus macrocyclic GBCAs.

RETENTION OF GADOLINIUM IN CENTRAL NERVOUS SYSTEM TISSUES

An initial study in 2010 found intracranial Gd retention among patients with brain tumors; however, these findings were attributed to disruption of the blood-brain barrier (BBB).[26] A subsequent study by Kanda and colleagues[27] in 2014 hypothesized that increasing T1 signal in the dentate nucleus and globus pallidus of patients exposed to GBCAs were caused by intracranial Gd retention. This hypothesis was confirmed by 2 studies that quantified elemental Gd in postmortem brain tissues of patients who received multiple doses of GBCAs over their lifetime.[5,6,27] Highest concentrations of Gd were observed in the dentate nucleus, with retention also confirmed in the globus pallidus, pons, and thalamus, with substantially lower levels of retention in other areas of the brain.[6] This preferential accumulation in specific neuroanatomic regions has been postulated to be a result of the chemical similarity between Gd and Ca, because these regions also happen to be locations where Ca also is preferentially accumulated in both physiologic and pathologic states.[28] Gd accumulation in neuronal tissues occurs in a dose-dependent manner in the setting of normal renal function and persists for years after GBCA exposure.[5] Subsequent studies have confirmed detectable levels of Gd after 1 dose of intravenous linear or macrocyclic GBCAs.[9] Significantly less Gd retention was observed, however, after macrocyclic versus linear agent exposure. These findings also have been observed in animal models.[7,8,10,29]

Transmission electron microscopy studies of neural tissues revealed that most of the Gd was

Table 1
Physical and chemical properties of GBCAs

| GBCA Name | | | | Physical & Chemical Properties | | | | |
Chemical	Trade	Structure	Ionicity	Protein Binding	r1	Log K$_{therm}$	Log K$_{cond}$	K$_{obs}$ (S^{-1})
Gadodiamide	Omniscan	Linear	Non-ionic	No	4.3	16.9	14.9	12.7
Gadoversetamide[a]	OptiMark[a]	Linear	Non-ionic	No	4.7	16.6	15.0	8.6
Gadopentetate dimeglumine[a]	Magnevist[a]	Linear	Ionic	No	4.1	22.5	18.4	0.58
Gadoxetic acid	Eovist	Linear	Ionic	Yes	6.9	23.5	18.7	0.16
Gadobenate dimeglumine	MultiHance	Linear	Ionic	Yes	7.9	22.6	18.4	0.41
Gadofosveset trisodium[a]	Ablavar[a]	Linear	Ionic	Yes	19.0	22.1	18.9	2.9×10^{-2}
Gadoteridol	ProHance	Macrocyclic	Non-ionic	No	4.1	23.8	17.1	2.6×10^{-4}
Gadobutrol	Gadavist	Macrocyclic	Non-ionic	No	4.1	21.8	14.7	2.8×10^{-5}
Gadoterate meglumine	Dotarem	Macrocyclic	Ionic	No	3.8	25.6	19.3	2.0×10^{-6}

Abbreviations: K$_{obs}$, kinetic lability, 0.1M HCl (sec^{-1}); Log K$_{cond}$, thermodynamic stability. pH 2 (M); Log K$_{therm}$, thermodynamic stability. pH 7.4 (M); r1, relaxivity (L/mmol*s).
[a] Withdrawn from the U.S. market.
Adapted from McDonald RJ, Levine D, Weinreb J, et al. Gadolinium Retention: A Research Roadmap from the 2018 NIH/ACR/RSNA Workshop on Gadolinium Chelates. Radiology 2018:181151; with permission.

localized to the endothelium of capillaries outside of the BBB. A much smaller fraction of Gd-enriched foci either circumvented or directly traversed the BBB and was detected in the neural interstitium and cellular organelles.[5,30,31] Gd deposits also have been observed in the nuclei of neuronal cells of the central nervous system (CNS),[30] raising additional concerns about the potential neurotoxicity of retained Gd.

Gd retention in CNS tissues has also been observed in patients with apparent intact BBB as well as in pediatric patients.[30,31] These findings challenge our understanding of the mechanisms of apparent permeability of the BBB to Gd.[32,33] The mechanism by which Gd transitions across the blood–cerebrospinal fluid (CSF) barrier and is retained in neural tissues is incompletely understood. There currently is no explicit evidence of Gd directly transgressing the intact BBB. Animal studies have shown that all GBCAs, regardless of class, enter the CSF from serum, and that neither GBCA structure nor physicochemical properties affect CSF penetration and distribution.[34] The presence of Gd in CSF has been verified in humans undergoing lumbar puncture after exposure to the macrocyclic GBCA gadobutrol. Gd clearance from CSF roughly approximated first-order kinetics, with detectable levels of Gd still present up to 30 days after initial GBCA administration.[35] The glymphatic system may be involved in the distribution and clearance of Gd from brain tissue.[36] Additional studies are needed to better understand how intravenously administered GBCAs result in Gd deposits in brain tissue.

RETENTION OF GADOLINIUM IN NON–CENTRAL NERVOUS SYSTEM TISSUES

Early biodistribution studies provided initial evidence of Gd retention in multiple animal tissues, including bone and liver.[23] The amount of retained Gd in organs varies by GBCA and appeared to be somewhat dependent on the lability and thermodynamic stability of the GBCA.[8,22,23] For example, 1 study demonstrated higher Gd levels in skin in gadodiamide-exposed rats and higher Gd levels in bone in gadopentetate-exposed rats.[37] Subsequent studies have shown, however, that stability and lability are not entirely predictive of retention, because Gd retention appears to differ between and within GBCA classes.[8] These observations underscore the complex biodistribution of GBCAs after intravenous injection in both animals and humans that is still poorly understood.

Multiple preclinical studies indicate that macrocyclic GBCAs have a faster washout from tissues compared with linear GBCAs.[38,39] In these

studies, it appears that a certain fraction of chronically retained Gd, particularly from linear GBCA administration, may be labile and/or may be bioconvertible to a mixture of both insoluble and more soluble forms of Gd. Longer-term washout data are needed at common time points to permit comparability between agents and classes.

Gd retention in the skin has been studied more extensively than other tissues and organs because of the efforts to understand the mechanisms underlying nephrogenic systemic fibrosis (NSF). The extent of Gd retention in skin again appears to depend on GBCA lability, suggesting a possible role for dechelation in long-term tissue retention.[22,23] Skin lesions associated with GBCA administration have been reported both in animal models and in human subjects.[37,40] These lesions are thought to represent an inflammatory, acute response rather than chronic Gd retention.[41] The presence of these lesions appears to be dose-dependent and typically are observed in animal models at supratherapeutic doses.[17,42]

Human autopsy studies have identified retained Gd in bone and skin samples of patients with normal renal function at least 2 years after GBCA administration,[9,17,43] with 1 study showing detectable levels of Gd in bone samples of patients 8 years after exposure.[16] This retention has been observed with both linear and macrocyclic GBCAs, with higher Gd levels observed after linear GBCA exposure. Gd levels in patient bone samples were much higher than those in skin or brain samples.[9] Gd retention in bone appears to depend on the GBCA, as gadodiamide-exposed patients had Gd levels in bone 4 times higher than gadoteridol-exposed patients.[43]

To the authors' knowledge, only 10 human studies of 133 total patients have been published to date that quantified Gd in tissues.[5,6,9,17,30,31,43–46] Many of these studies included patients exposed to multiple different GBCAs during their lifetime, such as a patient who was administered gadodiamide and gadoteridol for separate MR imaging examinations. Because Gd retention and washout have been shown to vary by GBCA, the inclusion of such patients confounds study results. No studies have been published quantifying Gd in other major organs of GBCA-exposed patients with normal renal function, such as the kidney, liver, heart, colon, and testes/ovaries. As such, the biodistribution of Gd in human organs and tissues is largely unknown, including whether there are differences between GBCAs, which organs demonstrate the highest amount of retained Gd, whether different organs have different rates of Gd washout, whether the chemical form of retained Gd varies between organs and tissues, and the cellular localization of Gd deposits in these organs and tissues. Such data are critical to understand the biodistribution and pharmacokinetics of retained Gd in patients and the potential biological and toxicologic effects chronically retained Gd deposits may have in vivo.

SPECIATION

Gd is retained in tissues in either a biologically inactive chelated form or potentially toxic dechelated forms, as described previously. Speciation studies have identified both insoluble and soluble forms of Gd, including intact GBCA molecules, in skin samples from NSF patients.[17,47,48] The chemical form of retained Gd appears to be GBCA specific, with intact forms of the macrocyclic gadoteridol detected in skin samples but not intact forms of gadodiamide.[48] Animal studies have identified Gd in the soluble fraction of homogenized brain tissue, likely as intact chelate, after macrocyclic GBCA exposure, whereas Gd was identified predominantly in the insoluble fraction, potentially bound to macromolecules (250–300 kDa), after linear GBCA exposure.[29,49–51] The chemical form of retained Gd appeared consistent in gadodiamide-exposed or gadoterate-exposed rats for up to 1 year after GBCA exposure.[50] Additional studies are needed to fully characterize the chemical forms of retained Gd in other organs and tissues.

TOXICOLOGY

The fate of the small fraction of administered GBCA that is not rapidly excreted is at the center of current concerns for chronic toxicity because (1) Gd has no known biological role in vivo and is known to have adverse biological effects[52–54]; (2) Gd plays a role in the development of NSF in some patients with long-term or high exposures[55–58]; and (3) some forms of residual Gd remain in tissues for years.[5,31] Thus, the small fraction of retained GBCA, or any products of its dissociation, may have potential for chronic toxic effects.

The acute toxic effects of rare earth metals have been observed in multiple organ systems (lung, liver, bowel, hematopoietic, and brain).[59–63] Manifestations of elemental forms of Gd toxicity include nephrotoxicity, hemotoxicity, and hepatotoxicity as well as neurotoxicity.[61] In contradistinction to free Gd, chelated forms of Gd found in GBCAs have been shown to be significantly less acutely cytotoxic in preclinical studies.[64]

To date, there has been no convincing evidence of chronic toxicity due to retained Gd in neural tissues introduced via intravenous administration of GBCAs. Studies of human brain tissues and animal studies have consistently failed to demonstrate histopathologic evidence of injury to neurons or the neural interstitium.[5,6,8,31,37,39] Potential nephrotoxicity, hepatoxicity, or toxicity of chronic Gd retention in other organs and tissues, however, has not been examined. Potential toxicity may depend on the total amount of retained Gd in the organ, or whether the retained Gd remains in its chelated form. Additional controlled studies are needed to evaluate the potential histopathologic changes in organs and tissues after GBCA exposure.

CLINICAL EFFECTS OF GADOLINIUM-BASED CONTRAST AGENTS EXPOSURE

The most well-known potential manifestation of chronic GBCA toxicity from standard clinical dosing is NSF, a rare but devastating condition defined by excessive collagen deposition in tissues that occurs weeks to years after GBCA exposure. NSF is thought to be a result of in vivo GBCA dissociation into a dechelated free form of Gd as a result of formation of more stable non-Gd:ligand complexes (eg, transmetallation). The resultant free Gd activates macrophages and circulating fibrocytes, leading to aberrant collagen deposition in connective tissues.[22,56] Fibrotic changes resulting from this collagen deposition have been seen in many tissues, but contractures in affected skin and muscle tissues primarily responsible for adverse symptoms, including swelling, tightening, and thickening of the skin and loss of joint flexibility.[55,56,65]

NSF is extremely uncommon, with approximately 613 verified cases reported to date and limited to a patient population with significant renal impairment.[66] Changes in clinical guidelines regarding the use of GBCAs in patients with severe renal insufficiency essentially have eradicated NSF. Furthermore, because the mechanisms of NSF are poorly understood, it is unknown if these effects are the result of acute exposure, chronically retained Gd forms in tissues, or a combination.

Apart from NSF, data linking GBCA exposure with chronic toxicologic findings among humans with normal renal function are scant and are limited to case reports or studies involving multiple or supratherapeutic GBCA doses.[3] More recently, patient-reported data have emerged from approximately 130 patients that may suggest neurologic, musculoskeletal, and connective tissue–related symptoms from GBCA exposure.[67–69] These clinical manifestations, termed *Gd deposition disease (GDD)*, have been reported to occur within minutes of GBCA administration. The FDA and other regulatory agencies and professional societies do not recognize this clinical entity as the causal relationship between GBCA exposure and development of these symptoms has not yet been established through rigorous scientific study. Notwithstanding, further research is needed to establish if this relationship is coincidental or causal and if GBCA exposure has other rare side effects not described or recognized in the medical literature.

CLINICAL IMPORTANCE OF GADOLINIUM RETENTION IN HUMANS

The critical question regarding Gd retention is whether it causes clinically meaningful effects. Hundreds of millions of GBCA doses have been administered in the United States for the past 3 decades without obvious clinical manifestations associated with Gd retention. Risk tolerance thresholds have been defined for acute reactions and the development of NSF, because these are confirmed and well-studied potential complications of GBCA exposure. There currently is no established risk tolerance threshold for chronic Gd retention. If Gd retention is associated with clinical harm, the harm is likely rare or occult for the vast majority of exposed patients.

To date, studies have identified approximately 130 patients, all with normal or minimally impaired renal function, who have reported effects that they associated with GBCA exposure.[68,69] Reported symptoms included chronic pain, fatigue, dermal changes, musculoskeletal disturbances, and cognitive and visual impairment. Some of these symptoms overlap with symptoms reported in patients with NSF. These effects have been reported to occur shortly (<24 hours to 1 month) after receiving only 1 GBCA dose and persist for months to years after exposure. This constellation of findings is termed GDD.[67]

There are major limitations, however, with these GDD studies. No control groups were included in these studies, and researchers were not blinded. Most GDD cases were self-reported and lacked details, such as the specific GBCA used, total GBCA dose, and the time to onset of symptoms. It is unknown what percentage of patients with retained Gd also develop symptoms. Importantly, the studies published to date have also not accounted for the obvious confounder of why these patients received GBCAs for their clinical care. For example, if a patient with an autoimmune disorder undergoes a GBCA-enhanced MR imaging examination and subsequently develops new joint pain, is this pain attributed to the underlying disorder, GBCA exposure, or both? Due to the these limitations, the causative association between these symptoms and retained Gd remains speculative. In 2017, the Medical Imaging Drugs Advisory Committee of the FDA concluded that no causal relationship between Gd retention and patient symptoms could be established but that further study was needed.[70]

Controlled preclinical studies examining the effects of GBCA exposure on neurologic functions have demonstrated mixed results, with several studies showing behavioral differences between GBCA-exposed and control animals.[71–73] In contrast, other studies did not report any differences between GBCA-exposed and control animals in a range of tests.[74,75] Additional studies are necessary to determine the reproducibility of these findings, examine other GBCAs, and examine the potential effects of GBCA exposure on other behavioral tests.

Studies of the potential clinical effects of GBCA exposure in humans also have shown mixed results. A longitudinal study comparing multiple sclerosis patients who received GBCAs to age-matched and sex-matched control patients found that increased signal intensity in the dentate nucleus in MS patients was associated with lower verbal fluency scores at neuropsychological testing.[76] The presence of neurologic disease, however, is a major confounder. A controlled large study of more than 1 million deliveries found that in utero contrast-enhanced MR imaging was associated with an increased risk of rheumatologic, inflammatory, and infiltrative skin conditions as well as an increased adjusted risk of stillbirth and neonatal death.[77] The study did not adjust, however, for the reason GBCA was administered during pregnancy. A study of patients with inflammatory bowel disease did not find evidence of brain functional changes in patients with visible T1 hyperintensity after exposure to gadodiamide; however, they did identify subtle nonsignificant changes in functional activation that may merit further investigation.[78]

Many questions remain if a causal link between GBCA exposure and GDD symptoms is confirmed. It is unknown whether the symptoms are caused by acute or semiacute processes resulting from exposure to, not long-term retention of, Gd. If studies confirm that these symptoms are caused by chronic retention of Gd, additional research will be needed to determine if these symptoms vary by GBCA type or GBCA class, if they are dose dependent, and if they are acute or delayed in onset. Studies should include as many GBCAs as are feasible, and GBCAs should be studied and reported as a class and individually. Suitable control groups must be included, and potentially confounding factors, such as preexisting clinical and laboratory parameters, time from last GBCA administration, and dosing schedule, should be considered. The specific signs, symptoms, and diseases to investigate are unclear. Studies should examine not only potential neurologic effects from Gd retention in brain tissue but also potential clinical effects from retention in other organs and tissues.

Chelation therapy has been proposed as a method for removing acutely retained or chronically retained Gd from tissues. A small uncontrolled study of 25 patients with self-reported GDD symptoms who underwent experimental chelation therapy had mixed effects in the relief of reported symptoms.[79] Gd levels decreased in liver tissues of GBCA-exposed pediatric patients after chelation therapy with deferoxamine mesylate.[80] Chelation therapy is associated, however, with known and potentially serious risks, whereas the correlation between Gd retention and clinical effects has not been confirmed. Larger, controlled studies examining the effectiveness of chelation therapy in removing Gd and relieving symptoms of GDD have yet to be performed. Notwithstanding, off-label chelation therapy continues to be performed on patients reporting GDD symptoms.

POTENTIAL AT-RISK POPULATIONS

There is emerging evidence that certain patient populations may be at increased risk of Gd retention, of possible Gd-mediated toxicity, and potentially of clinical symptoms associated with Gd retention.[3] These populations must be specifically studied, because clinical symptoms of Gd retention may be observed only in these groups compared with healthy adults.

Fetal, infant, and early childhood populations may be at increased risk from GBCA exposure due to their ongoing growth, development, and high cell turnover compared with adults, particularly in the CNS and bone. Pediatric patients are known to be at increased risk of metal toxicity in the brain and other organs due to their ongoing development. Furthermore, because pediatric patients receive GBCAs early in their lifetime and may retain Gd in tissues for their entire lives, they may be susceptible to other clinical effects compared with adults. One study showed that administration of GBCAs to pregnant nonhuman primates resulted in measurable Gd concentration in bone and other organs of offspring for at least

7 months.[81] Detectable Gd levels were observed in liver tissue of pediatric patients with concomitant iron overload amenable to chelation therapy with deferoxamine mesylate.[80] Skin lesions were observed exclusively in gadodiamide-exposed juvenile rats and higher levels of Gd in bone were found in juvenile rats compared with adult rats.[71]

Adults with certain comorbidities also may be at increased risk from GBCA exposure. Patients with decreased renal function have been shown to have reduced clearance of Gd,[18] possibly resulting in increased Gd retention in tissues and an increased risk of Gd-mediated toxicity and clinical symptoms. Several rat model studies have demonstrated higher levels of Gd in serum and multiple organs in rats with renal insufficiency compared to control animals.[82–84] Patients who develop osteoporosis, renal osteodystrophy, or hyperparathyroidism may be at risk of mobilization of Gd from bone. Patients with an immature or altered BBB may be predisposed to Gd retention in brain tissue. Finally, patients who are exposed to higher levels of iron, zinc, manganese, lanthanides, or copper may be at greater risk for transmetallation effects when exposed to a GBCA.[47,80,85,86] Future studies may uncover additional clinical conditions that increase Gd retention.

SUMMARY

GBCAs have been used clinically for more than 30 years; however, important information about GBCA biodistribution and tissue interactions remains unknown. Gd retention in several tissues, including bone, skin, and brain, appears to occur with all GBCAs, although the magnitude of observed retention is greater with linear GBCAs than with macrocyclic GBCAs. The extent, mechanism, chemical form, and clinical implications of chronic Gd retention for each GBCA have not been fully characterized in the general population or in potentially vulnerable populations. Additional studies are necessary to improve understanding of Gd retention and its clinical importance.

DISCLOSURE

J.S. McDonald and R.J. McDonald report research grants with GE Healthcare. R.J. McDonald report research grants with Bracco Imaging. J.S. McDonald and R.J. McDonald serve as scientific advisors for GE Healthcare.

REFERENCES

1. Caravan P, Ellison JJ, McMurry TJ, et al. Gadolinium(III) chelates as MRI contrast agents: structure,

dynamics, and applications. Chem Rev 1999;99(9): 2293–352.

2. Zhou Z, Lu ZR. Gadolinium-based contrast agents for magnetic resonance cancer imaging. Wiley Interdiscip Rev Nanomed Nanobiotechnol 2013;5(1): 1–18.

3. McDonald RJ, Levine D, Weinreb J, et al. Gadolinium retention: a research roadmap from the 2018 NIH/ACR/RSNA workshop on gadolinium chelates. Radiology 2018;289(2):517–34.

4. Balzer T. Presence of gadolinium (Gd) in the brain and body. Meeting of the Medical Imaging Drugs Advisory Committee (MIDAC): US Food and Drug Administration. September 8, 2017.

5. McDonald RJ, McDonald JS, Kallmes DF, et al. Intracranial gadolinium deposition after contrast-enhanced MR imaging. Radiology 2015;275(3): 772–82.

6. Kanda T, Fukusato T, Matsuda M, et al. Gadolinium-based contrast agent accumulates in the brain even in subjects without severe renal dysfunction: evaluation of autopsy brain specimens with inductively coupled plasma mass spectroscopy. Radiology 2015;276(1):228–32.

7. Bussi S, Coppo A, Botteron C, et al. Differences in gadolinium retention after repeated injections of macrocyclic MR contrast agents to rats. J Magn Reson Imaging 2018;47(3):746–52.

8. McDonald RJ, McDonald JS, Dai D, et al. Comparison of gadolinium concentrations within multiple rat organs after intravenous administration of linear versus macrocyclic gadolinium chelates. Radiology 2017;285(2):536–45.

9. Murata N, Gonzalez-Cuyar LF, Murata K, et al. Macrocyclic and other non-group 1 gadolinium contrast agents deposit low levels of gadolinium in brain and bone tissue: preliminary results from 9 patients with normal renal function. Invest Radiol 2016; 51(7):447–53.

10. Robert P, Lehericy S, Grand S, et al. T1-weighted hypersignal in the deep cerebellar nuclei after repeated administrations of gadolinium-based contrast agents in healthy rats: difference between linear and macrocyclic agents. Invest Radiol 2015; 50(8):473–80.

11. Agency EM. PRAC concludes assessment of gadolinium agents used in body scans and recommends regulatory actions, including suspension for some marketing authorisations EMA/157486/2017. Pharmacovigilance Risk Assessment Committee. 2017;EMA/157486/ 2017 Pharmacovigilance Risk Assessment Committee.

12. United States Food and Drug Administration. FDA briefing document: gadolinium retention after gadolinium based contrast magnetic resonance imaging in patients with normal renal function. White Oak (MD): U.S. Food and Drug Administration; 2017. Available at: https://www.fda.gov/downloads/AdvisoryCommittees/CommitteesMeetingMaterials/Drugs/MedicalImagingDrugsAdvisoryCommittee/UCM572848.pdf. Accessed July 27, 2020.

13. United States Food and Drug Administration. FDA Drug Safety Communication: FDA warns that gadolinium-based contrast agents (GBCAs) are retained in the body; requires new class warnings. White Oak (MD): U.S. Food and Drug Administration; 2017. Available at: https://www.fda.gov/Drugs/DrugSafety/ucm589213.htm. Accessed July 27, 2020.

14. Wedeking P, Kumar K, Tweedle MF. Dissociation of gadolinium chelates in mice: relationship to chemical characteristics. Magn Reson Imaging 1992; 10(4):641–8.

15. Tweedle MF. Gadolinium deposition: is it chelated or dissociated gadolinium? How can we tell? Magn Reson Imaging 2016;34(10):1377–82.

16. Darrah TH, Prutsman-Pfeiffer JJ, Poreda RJ, et al. Incorporation of excess gadolinium into human bone from medical contrast agents. Metallomics 2009;1(6):479–88.

17. Roberts DR, Lindhorst SM, Welsh CT, et al. High levels of gadolinium deposition in the skin of a patient with normal renal function. Invest Radiol 2016; 51(5):280–9.

18. Prybylski JP, Jay M. The impact of excess ligand on the retention of nonionic, linear gadolinium-based contrast agents in patients with various levels of renal dysfunction: a review and simulation analysis. Adv Chronic Kidney Dis 2017;24(3):176–82.

19. Di Gregorio E, Ferrauto G, Furlan C, et al. The issue of gadolinium retained in tissues: insights on the role of metal complex stability by comparing metal uptake in murine tissues upon the concomitant administration of lanthanum- and gadolinium-diethylentriamminopentaacetate. Invest Radiol 2018;53(3):167–72.

20. Lancelot E. Revisiting the pharmacokinetic profiles of gadolinium-based contrast agents: differences in long-term biodistribution and excretion. Invest Radiol 2016;51(11):691–700.

21. Semelka RC, Commander CW, Jay M, et al. Presumed gadolinium toxicity in subjects with normal renal function: a report of 4 cases. Invest Radiol 2016;51(10):661–5.

22. Pietsch H, Lengsfeld P, Jost G, et al. Long-term retention of gadolinium in the skin of rodents following the administration of gadolinium-based contrast agents. Eur Radiol 2009;19(6):1417–24.

23. Tweedle MF, Wedeking P, Kumar K. Biodistribution of radiolabeled, formulated gadopentetate, gadoteridol, gadoterate, and gadodiamide in mice and rats. Invest Radiol 1995;30(6):372–80.

24. Robert P, Frenzel T, Factor C, et al. Methodological aspects for preclinical evaluation of gadolinium presence in brain tissue: critical appraisal and suggestions for harmonization-a joint initiative. Invest Radiol 2018;53(9):499–517.

25. Jost G, Frenzel T, Boyken J, et al. Long-term excretion of gadolinium-based contrast agents: linear versus macrocyclic agents in an experimental rat model. Radiology 2019;290(2):340–8.

26. Xia D, Davis RL, Crawford JA, et al. Gadolinium released from MR contrast agents is deposited in brain tumors: in situ demonstration using scanning electron microscopy with energy dispersive X-ray spectroscopy. Acta Radiol 2010;51(10):1126–36.

27. Kanda T, Ishii K, Kawaguchi H, et al. High signal intensity in the dentate nucleus and globus pallidus on unenhanced T1-weighted MR images: relationship with increasing cumulative dose of a gadolinium-based contrast material. Radiology 2014;270(3):834–41.

28. Valdes Hernandez Mdel C, Maconick LC, Tan EM, et al. Identification of mineral deposits in the brain on radiological images: a systematic review. Eur Radiol 2012;22(11):2371–81.

29. Gianolio E, Bardini P, Arena F, et al. Gadolinium retention in the rat brain: assessment of the amounts of insoluble gadolinium-containing species and intact gadolinium complexes after repeated administration of gadolinium-based contrast agents. Radiology 2017;285(3):839–49.

30. McDonald JS, McDonald RJ, Jentoft ME, et al. Intracranial gadolinium deposition following gadodiamide-enhanced magnetic resonance imaging in pediatric patients: a case-control study. JAMA Pediatr 2017;171(7):705–7.

31. McDonald RJ, McDonald JS, Kallmes DF, et al. Gadolinium deposition in human brain tissues after contrast-enhanced MR imaging in adult patients without intracranial abnormalities. Radiology 2017;285(2):546–54.

32. Kanal E, Tweedle MF. Residual or retained gadolinium: practical implications for radiologists and our patients. Radiology 2015;275(3):630–4.

33. Montagne A, Toga AW, Zlokovic BV. Blood-brain barrier permeability and gadolinium: benefits and potential pitfalls in research. JAMA Neurol 2016;73(1):13–4.

34. Jost G, Frenzel T, Lohrke J, et al. Penetration and distribution of gadolinium-based contrast agents into the cerebrospinal fluid in healthy rats: a potential pathway of entry into the brain tissue. Eur Radiol 2017;27(7):2877–85.

35. Nehra AK, McDonald RJ, Bluhm AM, et al. Accumulation of gadolinium in human cerebrospinal fluid after gadobutrol-enhanced MR imaging: a prospective observational cohort study. Radiology 2018;288(2):416–23.

36. Taoka T, Jost G, Frenzel T, et al. Impact of the glymphatic system on the kinetic and distribution of gadodiamide in the rat brain: observations by dynamic MRI and effect of circadian rhythm on tissue gadolinium concentrations. Invest Radiol 2018;53(9):529–34.

37. Lohrke J, Frisk AL, Frenzel T, et al. Histology and gadolinium distribution in the rodent brain after the administration of cumulative high doses of linear and macrocyclic gadolinium-based contrast agents. Invest Radiol 2017;52(6):324–33.

38. Jost G, Frenzel T, Boyken J, et al. Long-term Excretion of Gadolinium-based Contrast Agents: Linear versus Macrocyclic Agents in an Experimental Rat Model. Radiology 2018;290(2):340–8.

39. Smith AP, Marino M, Roberts J, et al. Clearance of gadolinium from the brain with no pathologic effect after repeated administration of gadodiamide in healthy rats: an analytical and histologic study. Radiology 2017;282(3):743–51.

40. Abujudeh HH, Kaewlai R, Kagan A, et al. Nephrogenic systemic fibrosis after gadopentetate dimeglumine exposure: case series of 36 patients. Radiology 2009;253(1):81–9.

41. Pietsch H, Raschke M, Ellinger-Ziegelbauer H, et al. The role of residual gadolinium in the induction of nephrogenic systemic fibrosis-like skin lesions in rats. Invest Radiol 2011;46(1):48–56.

42. Christensen KN, Lee CU, Hanley MM, et al. Quantification of gadolinium in fresh skin and serum samples from patients with nephrogenic systemic fibrosis. J Am Acad Dermatol 2011;64(1):91–6.

43. White GW, Gibby WA, Tweedle MF. Comparison of Gd(DTPA-BMA) (Omniscan) versus Gd(HP-DO3A) (ProHance) relative to gadolinium retention in human bone tissue by inductively coupled plasma mass spectroscopy. Invest Radiol 2006;41(3):272–8.

44. Fingerhut S, Sperling M, Holling M, et al. Gadolinium-based contrast agents induce gadolinium deposits in cerebral vessel walls, while the neuropil is not affected: an autopsy study. Acta Neuropathol 2018;136(1):127–38.

45. Kiviniemi A, Gardberg M, Ek P, et al. Gadolinium retention in gliomas and adjacent normal brain tissue: association with tumor contrast enhancement and linear/macrocyclic agents. Neuroradiology 2019;61(5):535–44.

46. Roberts DR, Welsh CA, LeBel DP 2nd, et al. Distribution map of gadolinium deposition within the cerebellum following GBCA administration. Neurology 2017;88(12):1206–8.

47. Abraham JL, Thakral C, Skov L, et al. Dermal inorganic gadolinium concentrations: evidence for in vivo transmetallation and long-term persistence in nephrogenic systemic fibrosis. Br J Dermatol 2008;158(2):273–80.

48. Birka M, Wentker KS, Lusmoller E, et al. Diagnosis of nephrogenic systemic fibrosis by means of elemental bioimaging and speciation analysis. Anal Chem 2015;87(6):3321–8.

49. Frenzel T, Apte C, Jost G, et al. Quantification and assessment of the chemical form of residual gadolinium in the brain after repeated administration of gadolinium-based contrast agents: comparative study in rats. Invest Radiol 2017;52(7):396–404.

50. Robert P, Fingerhut S, Factor C, et al. One-year retention of gadolinium in the brain: comparison of gadodiamide and gadoterate meglumine in a rodent model. Radiology 2018;288(2):424–33.

51. Strzeminska I, Factor C, Robert P, et al. Long-term evaluation of gadolinium retention in rat brain after single injection of a clinically relevant dose of gadolinium-based contrast agents. Invest Radiol 2020;55(3):138–43.

52. Feng L, Xiao H, He X, et al. Neurotoxicological consequence of long-term exposure to lanthanum. Toxicol Lett 2006;165(2):112–20.

53. Sherry AD, Caravan P, Lenkinski RE. Primer on gadolinium chemistry. J Magn Reson Imaging 2009; 30(6):1240–8.

54. Muldoon LL, Neuwelt EA. Dose-dependent neurotoxicity (seizures) due to deposition of gadolinium-based contrast agents in the central nervous system. Radiology 2015;277(3):925–6.

55. Boyd AS, Zic JA, Abraham JL. Gadolinium deposition in nephrogenic fibrosing dermopathy. J Am Acad Dermatol 2007;56(1):27–30.

56. Grobner T, Prischl FC. Gadolinium and nephrogenic systemic fibrosis. Kidney Int 2007;72(3):260–4.

57. Thakral C, Alhariri J, Abraham JL. Long-term retention of gadolinium in tissues from nephrogenic systemic fibrosis patient after multiple gadolinium-enhanced MRI scans: case report and implications. Contrast Media Mol Imaging 2007;2(4):199–205.

58. Rofsky NM, Sherry AD, Lenkinski RE. Nephrogenic systemic fibrosis: a chemical perspective. Radiology 2008;247(3):608–12.

59. Wermuth PJ, Jimenez SA. Induction of a type I interferon signature in normal human monocytes by gadolinium-based contrast agents: comparison of linear and macrocyclic agents. Clin Exp Immunol 2014;175(1):113–25.

60. Rim KT, Koo KH, Park JS. Toxicological evaluations of rare earths and their health impacts to workers: a literature review. Saf Health Work 2013;4(1):12–26.

61. Rogosnitzky M, Branch S. Gadolinium-based contrast agent toxicity: a review of known and proposed mechanisms. Biometals 2016;29(3):365–76.

62. Ramalho J, Castillo M, AlObaidy M, et al. High signal intensity in globus pallidus and dentate nucleus on unenhanced T1-weighted MR images: evaluation of two linear gadolinium-based contrast agents. Radiology 2015;276(3):836–44.

63. Xia Q, Feng X, Huang H, et al. Gadolinium-induced oxidative stress triggers endoplasmic reticulum stress in rat cortical neurons. J Neurochem 2011; 117(1):38–47.

64. Nunn AD, Wedeking P, Marinelli E, et al. Toxicity of gadolinium chelates in rodents. Acad Radiol 1996; 3(Suppl 2):S333–5.

65. Marckmann P, Skov L, Rossen K, et al. Nephrogenic systemic fibrosis: suspected causative role of gadodiamide used for contrast-enhanced magnetic resonance imaging. J Am Soc Nephrol 2006;17(9): 2359–62.

66. Krefting I. Gadolinium retention following gadolinium based contrast agent MRIs: brain and other organs. September 8, 2017 Meeting of the Medical Imaging Drugs Advisory Committee (MIDAC): US Food and Drug Administration. September 8, 2017.

67. Semelka RC, Ramalho J, Vakharia A, et al. Gadolinium deposition disease: initial description of a disease that has been around for a while. Magn Reson Imaging 2016;34(10):1383–90.

68. Burke LM, Ramalho M, AlObaidy M, et al. Self-reported gadolinium toxicity: a survey of patients with chronic symptoms. Magn Reson Imaging 2016;34(8):1078–80.

69. Williams S, Grimm H. Gadolinium toxicity a survey of the chronic effects of retained gadolinium from contrast MRIs. Available at: https://gdtoxicity.files. wordpress.com/2014/09/gd-symptom-survey.pdf. Accessed July 27, 2020.

70. Food and Drug Administration Center for Drug Evaluation and Research MIDACM. Transcript: Friday, September 8, 2017, 7:30 a.m. to 4:10 p.m. FDA White Oak Campus, White Oak Conference Center, Building 31, The Great Room, Silver Spring, Maryland. 2017. Available at: https://www.fda.gov/downloads/ AdvisoryCommittees/CommitteesMeetingMaterials/ Drugs/MedicalImagingDrugsAdvisoryCommittee/ UCM584442.pdf. Accessed July 27, 2020.

71. Fretellier N, Granottier A, Rasschaert M, et al. Does age interfere with gadolinium toxicity and presence in brain and bone tissues?: A comparative gadoterate versus gadodiamide study in juvenile and adult rats. Invest Radiol 2019;54(2):61–71.

72. Inc. BHP. Gadolinium Based Contrast Agents (GBCAs). United States Food and Drug Administration - Medical Imaging Drugs Advisory Committee (MIDAC). September 8, 2017.

73. Khairinisa MA, Takatsuru Y, Amano I, et al. The effect of perinatal gadolinium-based contrast agents on adult mice behavior. Invest Radiol 2018;53(2): 110–8.

74. Bussi S, Penard L, Bonafe R, et al. Non-clinical assessment of safety and gadolinium deposition after cumulative administration of gadobenate dimeglumine (MultiHance((R))) to neonatal and juvenile rats. Regul Toxicol Pharmacol 2018;92:268–77.

75. Giorgi H, Ammerman J, Briffaux JP, et al. Non-clinical safety assessment of gadoterate meglumine (Dotarem((R))) in neonatal and juvenile rats. Regul Toxicol Pharmacol 2015;73(3):960–70.

76. Forslin Y, Shams S, Hashim F, et al. Retention of gadolinium-based contrast agents in multiple sclerosis: retrospective analysis of an 18-year longitudinal study. AJNR Am J Neuroradiol 2017;38(7): 1311–6.

77. Ray JG, Vermeulen MJ, Bharatha A, et al. Association between MRI exposure during pregnancy and fetal and childhood outcomes. JAMA 2016;316(9): 952–61.

78. Mallio CA, Piervincenzi C, Gianolio E, et al. Absence of dentate nucleus resting-state functional connectivity changes in nonneurological patients with gadolinium-related hyperintensity on T1 -weighted images. J Magn Reson Imaging 2019;50(2):445–55.

79. Semelka RC, Ramalho M, Jay M, et al. Intravenous calcium-/zinc-diethylene triamine penta-acetic acid in patients with presumed gadolinium deposition disease: a preliminary report on 25 patients. Invest Radiol 2018;53(6):373–9.

80. Maximova N, Gregori M, Zennaro F, et al. Hepatic gadolinium deposition and reversibility after contrast agent-enhanced MR Imaging of pediatric hematopoietic stem cell transplant recipients. Radiology 2016;281(2):418–26.

81. Oh KY, Roberts VH, Schabel MC, et al. Gadolinium chelate contrast material in pregnancy: fetal biodistribution in the nonhuman primate. Radiology 2015;276(1):110–8.

82. Kartamihardja AA, Nakajima T, Kameo S, et al. Impact of impaired renal function on gadolinium retention after administration of gadolinium-based contrast agents in a mouse model. Invest Radiol 2016;51(10):655–60.

83. Rasschaert M, Idee JM, Robert P, et al. Moderate renal failure accentuates T1 signal enhancement in the deep cerebellar nuclei of gadodiamide-treated rats. Invest Radiol 2017;52(5):255–64.

84. Delfino R, Biasotto M, Candido R, et al. Gadolinium tissue deposition in the periodontal ligament of mice with reduced renal function exposed to Gd-based contrast agents. Toxicol Lett 2019;301: 157–67.

85. Ghio AJ, Soukup JM, Dailey LA, et al. Gadolinium exposure disrupts iron homeostasis in cultured cells. J Biol Inorg Chem 2011;16(4):567–75.

86. Greenberg SA. Zinc transmetallation and gadolinium retention after MR imaging: case report. Radiology 2010;257(3):670–3.

Magnetic Resonance Safety: Pregnancy and Lactation

Jason T. Little, MD, Candice A. Bookwalter, MD, PhD*

KEYWORDS

- MRI • Safety • Pregnancy • Lactation • Gadolinium • GBCA • Ferumoxytol

KEY POINTS

- Biologic effects of the static magnetic field, radiofrequency energy deposition, and acoustic injury represent small risk to the fetus and are without known consequences.
- There have been no reported cases of NSF after in utero GBCA exposure; however, an increased risk of a rheumatological, inflammatory, or infiltrative skin conditions has been reported.
- Ultrasmall paramagnetic iron oxide particles such as ferumoxytol may be an alternative intravenous contrast agent for the pregnant patient and may not cross the placenta.
- Less than 1% of 0.04% of the intravenous dose of GBCA is excreted into breast milk; therefore no interruption of breast feeding is recommended.
- It is unknown whether USPIOs are excreted into breast milk.

INTRODUCTION

Utilization of MRI in the United States has markedly increased over the past few decades, with the number of scans per population approximately quadrupling from 1996 to 2016.[1] Additionally, the number of clinical indications for noncontrast MRI of a pregnant woman meeting American College of Radiology (ACR) appropriateness criteria has expanded, and includes acute abdominal or pelvic pain, suspected pancreaticobiliary disease, new-onset severe headache, new-onset atraumatic seizures, newly diagnosed cancer, and further evaluation of fetal anomalies detected by ultrasound or laboratory analysis, among other indications.[2,3]

For the attending radiologist assessing the risks and benefits of magnetic resonance scanning of a pregnant patient, the initial consideration is whether the information from MRI is likely to benefit the mother and/or fetus. Determination of whether evaluation can be adequately made with another imaging modality such as ultrasound and whether magnetic resonance scanning may be safely delayed until after the completion of the pregnancy is important and may circumvent potential risks to the fetus.

Specific risks to the fetus during MRI can be divided into 4categories: (1) biological effects of the static field, (2) radiofrequency (RF) energy deposition, (3) acoustic injury ,and (4) intravenous (IV) contrast. The first 3 categories are inherent to the magnetic resonance environment and may be mitigated but not eliminated. However, MRI examinations may be performed with or without IV contrast. The most commonly used IV contrast agents are gadolinium-based contrast agents (GBCAs) and less commonly ultrasmall paramagnetic iron oxide particles (USPIOs). Both GBCAs and USPIOs introduce additional maternal and fetal risks.

MAGNETIC RESONANCE SAFETY CONSIDERATIONS DURING PREGNANCY
Static Field

Biologic effects of the static magnetic field potentially inducing teratogenesis or fetal demise have been theorized, particularly during the first trimester. Various investigations with animal

Department of Radiology, Mayo Clinic, 200 First Street Southwest, Rochester, MN 55905, USA
* Corresponding author.
E-mail address: Bookwalter.Candice@mayo.edu

Magn Reson Imaging Clin N Am 28 (2020) 509–516
https://doi.org/10.1016/j.mric.2020.06.002
1064-9689/20/© 2020 Elsevier Inc. All rights reserved.

mri.theclinics.com

models have shown detectable effects from the static field. Studies of frog embryos and zebrafish eggs exposed to ultrahigh static magnetic fields (9–16T) for long durations (at least 24 hours) showed plausible mechanisms of developmental injury, but it is questionable whether the results of these animal studies are applicable to magnetic resonance scanning of human fetuses under ordinary clinical conditions.[4,5] Multiple retrospective studies of children who had been exposed to MRI in utero provide evidence that the risk of teratogenesis and/or miscarriage is extremely low and likely negligible. A 2015 retrospective study of 1737 children whose mothers had undergone MRI during the first trimester of gestation showed no statistically significant increase in adverse outcomes such as fetal demise, congenital abnormality, neoplasm, or vision or hearing loss.[6] A 2019 retrospective study of 81 neonates exposed in utero to 3T MRI showed no adverse effects at the higher field strength.[7]

Radiofrequency Energy Deposition

RF energy deposition is known to cause tissue heating. This is potentially problematic as there is a theoretic risk to the fetus if maternal body temperature increases by 2° to 2.5° C for a duration greater than 30 to 60 minutes. The fetus has limited capacity to regulate its own temperature, and spontaneous abortion has been reported in situations causing elevated maternal temperature like maternal fever and hot tub use.[8] Tissue heating by RF pulses has been shown to have a highly heterogeneous spatial distribution throughout the body, making prediction of heating of a discrete volume within the body extremely difficult.[9] One recent study using body models from 4 pregnant women observed significant variation in estimated fetal peak local specific absorption rate (SAR) with changes in maternal position within the scanner and fetal position within the uterus.[10] Therefore, the International Electrotechnical Commission (IEC) mandates a limit for pregnant patients of whole-body SAR of 2 W/kg, or normal operating mode, which is expected to result in a maximum temperature increase of 0.5° C over a 30-minute period.[11,12]

Even with this conservative approach, hot spots can theoretically occur in focal locations within the body, despite adhering to average whole-body SAR limits. In practice, RF tissue heating is greatest at the periphery of the body and minimal at the center, where the fetus is located. Experiments with phantom models and animal models have confirmed this distribution of energy. A study scanning gravid miniature pigs at 3T found that low-SAR protocols lasting less than 30 minutes resulted in less than 1° C temperature increase in the pig fetus. High-SAR protocols lasting longer than an hour did induce a temperature increase of 2.5° C, which is considered the upper limit of allowable temperature increase before tissue damage occurs.[13]

Thermal load estimated by SAR should not be confused with the phenomenon of focal burns.[14] Burns sustained during MRI are rare, and many reported incidents occur in the presence of conducting materials such as monitoring equipment, tattoos, or permanent cosmetics containing metallic pigments.[15] Focal burns can also occur at locations with skin-to-skin contact (eg, fingertips or calves) completing a circuit loop for induced current.[16,17] Focal burns are not specific to the pregnant patient, and the same precautions used for the nonpregnant patient should be implemented to avoid the risk of focal burns.

A special situation that may be rarely encountered is failure of an intrauterine device (IUD), where the IUD is retained but displaced and an intrauterine pregnancy results.[18] The most common IUDs are either nonmetallic, consisting of plastic and designed to release progesterone, or metallic and made with copper. Nonmetallic IUDs should not pose heating risk during magnetic resonance scanning. Copper is not ferromagnetic, and copper IUDs are generally magnetic resonance conditional with low risk for deflection, torque, or RF heating.[19] However, rarely stainless steel IUDs (eg, the Chinese ring) may be encountered and have been shown to induce artifacts and are categorized as unsafe in the magnetic resonance environment because of magnetic dislocation and torque.[20] If both an intrauterine pregnancy and intrauterine device are present, it is important to determine the type of IUD present to assess the risks to the fetus.

Tools at the disposal of the radiologist and technologist to mitigate the risk of tissue heating include scanning in normal operating mode to adhere to whole-body SAR limits, or scanning at 1.5 T instead of 3T, as doubling the magnetic field strength will increase the SAR by 4 times if other parameters are unchanged. RF energy deposition is not considered by the ACR or the American College of Obstetricians and Gynecologists (ACOG) to be a significant risk to the fetus at either 1.5 T or 3T assuming adherence to appropriate guidelines.[21,22]

Acoustic Noise

Acoustic noise generated by the magnetic resonance scanner represents another important consideration for fetal safety. Human fetuses have been shown to react to noises from outside the mother as early as 19 to 20 weeks of gestation.[23] By 24 weeks of gestation, the fetal ear has developed and can be injured by excessive noise.[15]

Time-dependent currents in gradient coils interact with the static magnetic field to produce strong Lorentz forces in the coils, resulting in microscopic vibrations capable of generating up to 140 dB of sound pressure (maximum allowable level established by the US Food and Drug Administration [FDA] for an MRI system).[24] Because this level of noise can potentially inflict permanent hearing loss, patients undergoing MRI are required to wear ear protection. The maternal tissue surrounding the fetus was estimated by 1 study to reduce sound pressure by approximately 30 dB.[25] However, another study performed in women in active labor showed a maximum reduction by only 10 dB, suggesting that factors such as amniotic fluid levels and possibly maternal and fetal positioning can affect the degree of sound attenuation.[26] The American Academy of Pediatrics recommends an upper limit of 90 dB, with risk of permanent hearing loss increasing above this level.[27] This upper limit of 90 dB is likely observed under ordinary scanning conditions in utero even in the presence of maternal tissue sound dampening.

Several studies evaluating for acoustic injury in children exposed to MRI in utero have suggested that, in clinical conditions, the risk is negligible. A 2010 study of 103 neonates exposed to 1.5 T MRI during the second and third trimesters of gestation showed no substantial risk of hearing impairment.[28] A 2015 study of 751 neonates who had undergone MRI in utero showed no adverse effects on neonatal hearing.[29] A 2019 study of 340 infants exposed to 3T MRI in utero also showed no evidence of hearing loss.[30]

Gadolinium-Based Contrast Agents

Gadolinium is toxic in its unbound form; however when tightly bound to a ligand, (GBCAs) are nontoxic and are used in approximately 30% to 45% of MRI examinations.[31] In a nonpregnant patient, indications for GBCAs include a multitude of conditions including epilepsy, multiple sclerosis, neoplasm (central nervous system or elsewhere in the body), and many more indications. Despite this widespread use in the general population, there are several special considerations for GBCA use during pregnancy with regard to maternal and fetal safety. Each case should be reviewed to determine whether IV contrast is necessary to answer the clinical question and

whether the potential benefits outweigh the risks. Potential benefits of contrast enhanced MRI in pregnancy have been described in the literature for accurate diagnosis of placenta accreta spectrum disorders[32–35] and ischemic/nonischemic cardiac disease[36] where maternal and/or fetal management may be altered by imaging findings.

Maternal gadolinium-based contrast agent short- and long-term risks

If a GBCA is given to a pregnant or lactating patient, the same general short-term and long-term risks apply compared with the general population. There areno data in the literature to suggest that these long-term or short-term risks are increased for a pregnant or lactating patient.

Short-term risks include allergic reactions and nonallergic reactions (eg, sneezing, nausea, and vomiting). However, there are several unique potential contrast reaction symptoms in the pregnant patient that are considered severe reactions, including nonreassuring fetal status (ie, recurrent late decelerations or prolonged fetal bradycardia on fetal heart tracing) and preterm labor.[37,38] GBCA reactions in a pregnant patient should be treated similarly to a nonpregnant patient with a few modifications.[37] Left lateral tilt positioning of the pregnant patient is recommended during treatment of severe reactions to improve blood return via the inferior vena cava. Additionally, in the setting of hypotension, maintaining systolic blood pressure greater than 90 mm Hg or greater than 80% of baseline systolic blood pressure is important to ensure adequate perfusion to the placenta.[39] A pregnant patient with a prior history of contrast reaction to GBCAs, and for whom the benefits of GBC- enhanced MRI outweigh the risks, can receive allergy premedication per ACR guidelines.[2,40] Note that both diphenhydramine and prednisone cross the placenta. There is a possible association between first trimester corticosteroid use and oral clefts, as well as potential for adrenal insufficiency or immunosuppression in newborns.[2]

Long-term risks include nephrogenic systemic fibrosis (NSF)[41–43] and retained intracranial gadolinium.[44,45]

NSF was first described in 2000 and subsequently in 2006 connected with IV administration of GBCA. NSF is a rare, debilitating, and ultimately fatal disease causing skin thickening and organ failure with only thousands of confirmed cases worldwide and typically occurring in patients with impaired renal function. No cases of NSF have been reported in a pregnant patient or after in utero exposure.[46]

Retained intracranial Gd was first described as observed T1 shortening predominantly in the globus pallidus and dentate nucleus and subsequently confirmed in autopsy patients as Gd.[44] Retained Gd has subsequently been demonstrated in other parts of the body, including the skin and bone marrow, but no clinical manifestation has been confirmed as a result of this retained Gd.[47–50]

Fetal risk of in utero gadolinium-based contrast agent exposure

Chelated gadolinium has been shown to cross the placenta and enter the fetal circulation.[22,51,52] The GBCA is filtered by the fetal kidneys and excreted into the amniotic fluid. From the amniotic fluid, the GBCA may be reabsorbed into maternal circulation and/or be reabsorbed by the fetus from the gastrointestinal (GI) tract after swallowing amniotic fluid.[53,54] If reabsorbed by the fetal GI tract, the GBCA is re-excreted via the fetal kidneys back to the amniotic fluid. There is a poorly understood, theoretic risk of disassociation of the Gd molecule and chelate due to this prolonged exposure via this recirculation mechanism.[2] One animal study found residual fetal gadolinium with the highest concentration in the kidney at 21 and 45 hours after administration.[55] For reference, the maternal plasma half-life is approximately 2 hours, with nearly the entire bloodstream cleared within 24 hours in a patient with normal renal function.

There are no adequate studies evaluating the adverse effects of in utero exposure to GBCAs in people; however, animal studies have shown adverse effects on the fetus at high or repeat doses.[56] Of note, only 23 cases of NSF have been reported in children, and none have been under the age of 6 years.[2]

A single study evaluated infant and childhood outcomes in 397 in utero GBCA-exposed pregnancies out of 1.4 million pregnancies in Ontario.[6] Although there was no statistically significant increase in risk for NSF-like conditions, there was an increased risk (1.36-fold increased risk compared with women who did not undergo an MRI during pregnancy) of a broad set of rheumatological, inflammatory, or infiltrative skin conditions including arthritis, vasculitis, bone disorder, dermatitis, or connective tissues calcification. There was also an increased risk for stillbirth and neonatal death (3.70-fold increased risk). Additional studies are needed to replicate these findings and address several limitations of the study including small number of exposed pregnancies, insufficient power to compare enhanced and unenhanced MRI, and lack of control for the reason for MRI examination.

Nongadolinium-Based Contrast Agents

Ferumoxytol is an ultrasmall paramagnetic iron oxide (USPIO) agent that is approved by the FDA for iron replacement therapy for anemia in adult patients with chronic kidney disease. Ferumoxytol has also been described as an IV MRI contrast agent.[57,58] USPIO agents cause regional T1 and T2* shortening and can be given as a rapid bolus or long infusion. Long infusions have been shown to have fewer adverse reactions. The most common adverse reactions are nausea, dizziness, and diarrhea,[57,59] but more serious reactions including hypotension and anaphylaxis have been reported.[60,61] There are no data to suggest that the risks of maternal adverse reactions are different in pregnancy. Maternal reactions to ferumoxytol should be treated the same as GBCAs.

The intravascular half-life is approximately 14 to 15 hours; however, USPIO agents are cleared by macrophage uptake and the reticuloendothelial system, and can take longer than 3 to 11 months.[62] The effects on the fetus of elevated iron content in the maternal body are unknown.

There are no studies of ferumoxytol toxicity in pregnant women. In large, maternally toxic doses 13 to 15 times the human dose, ferumoxytol was shown to cause fetal malformations and decreases fetal weight in animal studies.[63] It has been suggested that ferumoxytol may not transport directly into fetal circulation given its large size of 30 nm (for reference, Gd 0.4 nm).[64] A recent study by Zhu and colleagues[65] looked at R2* and tissue susceptibility as a marker of iron deposition after administration of ferumoxytol in 11 nonhuman primates. This study found no evidence of iron deposition in fetal tissues and no evidence of iron in the amniotic fluid after maternal ferumoxytol administration. Increased R2* and tissue susceptibility were seen in the placenta on days 0 to 1, but not later, suggesting blood pool enhancement rather than deposition. Increased R2* was seen in the maternal liver for more than 3 weeks, similar to prior reported clearance.[57]

Because the risk of in utero exposure to ferumoxytol is largely unknown, the ACOG recommends use of GBCA if a contrast agent is deemed clinically necessary. ACR has no published recommendation on USPIO agents.

Screening

A utilization study by Bird and colleagues[66] showed a 4.3-fold greater prevalence of GBCA use during the first trimester compared with the second trimester and a 5.1-fold greater prevalence compared with the third trimester. This greater prevalence in the first trimester may suggest that there is a failure of screening in the first trimester. This highlights the importance of appropriate and thorough screening methods.

Identifying a pregnant patient is a unique challenge, as patients may not be aware of their pregnancies, particularly at an early gestational age prior to implantation when a pregnancy test may be falsely negative.[67] ACR recommends screening women of reproductive age for pregnancy before any MRI examination.[2] Appropriate screening for pregnancy should be a multistep process, including written safety screening form, direct questioning by technologist, prominently displayed signs, and pregnancy testing, when appropriate. When MRI is deemed to be clinically necessary during pregnancy, the patient should initially be screened as any other patient undergoing MRI, evaluating for implanted medical devices and foreign bodies.[68] In their institution, the authors test for pregnancy in appropriate patients undergoing MRI, screen pregnant patients before MRI as per usual, verify that the clinical question cannot be answered using another imaging modality, and scan using normal operating mode.

MAGNETIC RESONANCE SAFETY CONSIDERATIONS DURING LACTATION

Less than 0.04% of an intravascular dose of a GBCA is excreted into breastmilk within the first 24 hours following administration. Subsequently, less than 1% of that dose will be absorbed by the infant's GI tract.[69] Given this low dose and therefore low risk to the nursing infant, both the ACR and ACOG recommend no interruption of breast feeding following GBCA administration.

In contrast, it is not known if ferumoxytol is excreted into human breast milk. The FDA suggests weighing the importance of ferumoxytol to the mother and the known benefits of nursing.[63] The ACR and ACOG have no published recommendation on use of ferumoxytol in a lactating patient. It is noteworthy that ferumoxytol has been given to pediatric patients with no known long-term adverse effects.[70–73]

SUMMARY

MRI can be an important diagnostic tool for maternal and fetal imaging of the pregnant patient. Although there are limited studies on the risks of MRI exposure in utero, there are no known adverse effects related to the static field, RF energy deposition, or acoustic noise. To mitigate heating risk caused by RF energy deposition, MRI should be performed with a whole-body SAR limit of 2 W/kg or normal operating mode.

The ACR position on MRI of pregnant patients is that noncontrast MRI can be performed in all trimesters if deemed clinically necessary. The official position of ACOG is that noncontrast MRI has not been associated with known adverse fetal effects.

Given the limited information regarding safety of GBCA on the fetus, the ACR recommends GBCA use only if their use is considered critical and the potential benefits outweigh the risks to the fetus. The ACR recommends using one of the agents believed to be low risk for the development of NSF (Group II agents) and given in the lowest possible dose to achieve diagnostic results. No consensus recommendation is available regarding USPIO contrast agents in pregnancy; however, animal studies suggest that USPIOs may not cross the placenta and may have a favorable safety profile for the fetus.

For pregnant patients, each case should be reviewed by the referring physician and radiologist, verifying that the information gained from an MRI examination cannot be obtained by another means with less risk, the information is needed to care for the patient and/or fetus during the pregnancy, and waiting until the patient is no longer pregnant would not be prudent. Determination should be made whether IV contrast is necessary to answer the clinical question and again whether the potential benefits outweigh the risks.

DISCLOSURE

The authors have nothing to disclose.

REFERENCES

1. OECD. Magnetic resonance imaging (MRI) exams (indicator) 2020. https://doi.org/10.1787/1d89353f-en. Accessed August 4, 2020.
2. ACR. ACR appropriateness criteria. 2018. Available at: https://www.acr.org/Clincal-Resources/ACR-Appropriateness-Criteria. Accessed January 31, 2020.
3. Mervak BM, Altun E, McGinty KA, et al. MRI in pregnancy: Indications and practical considerations. J Magn Reson Imaging 2019;49(3):621–31.
4. Denegre JM, Valles JM Jr, Lin K, et al. Cleavage planes in frog eggs are altered by strong magnetic fields. Proc Natl Acad Sci U S A 1998;95(25):14729–32.
5. Ge S, Li J, Huang D, et al. Strong static magnetic field delayed the early development of zebrafish. Open Biol 2019;9(10):190137.
6. Ray JG, Vermeulen MJ, Bharatha A, et al. Association between MRI exposure during pregnancy and fetal and childhood outcomes. JAMA 2016;316(9):952–61.
7. Chartier AL, Bouvier MJ, McPherson DR, et al. The safety of maternal and fetal MRI at 3 T. AJR Am J Roentgenol 2019;213(5):1170–3.

8. Ziskin MC, Morrissey J. Thermal thresholds for tera-togenicity, reproduction, and development. Int J Hyperthermia 2011;27(4):374–87.

9. Chansakul T, Young GS. Neuroimaging in pregnant women. Semin Neurol 2017;37(6):712–23.

10. Abaci Turk E, Yetisir F, Adalsteinsson E, et al. Individual variation in simulated fetal SAR assessed in multiple body models. Magn Reson Med 2020;83(4):1418–28.

11. IEC. Medical electrical equipment-part 2–33: particular requirements for the basic safety and essential performance of magnetic resonance equipment for medical diagnosis. International Electrotechnical Commission; 2010. 60601-2-33.

12. Murbach M, Neufeld E, Samaras T, et al. Pregnant women models analyzed for RF exposure and temperature increase in 3T RF shimmed birdcages. Magn Reson Med 2017;77(5):2048–56.

13. Cannie MM, De Keyzer F, Van Laere S, et al. Potential heating effect in the gravid uterus by using 3-T MR imaging protocols: experimental study in miniature pigs. Radiology 2016;279(3):754–61.

14. Greenberg TD, Hoff MN, Gilk TB, et al. ACR guidance document on MR safe practices: updates and critical information 2019. J Magn Reson Imaging 2020;51(2):331–8.

15. Ciet P, Litmanovich DE. MR safety issues particular to women. Magn Reson Imaging Clin N Am 2015;23(1):59–67.

16. Knopp MV, Essig M, Debus J, et al. Unusual burns of the lower extremities caused by a closed conducting loop in a patient at MR imaging. Radiology 1996;200(2):572–5.

17. Tsai LL, Grant AK, Mortele KJ, et al. A practical guide to MR imaging safety: what radiologists need to know. Radiographics 2015;35(6):1722–37.

18. Heinemann K, Reed S, Moehner S, et al. Comparative contraceptive effectiveness of levonorgestrel-releasing and copper intrauterine devices: the European Active Surveillance Study for Intrauterine Devices. Contraception 2015;91(4):280–3.

19. Correia L, Ramos AB, Machado AI, et al. Magnetic resonance imaging and gynecological devices. Contraception 2012;85(6):538–43.

20. Bussmann S, Luechinger R, Froehlich JM, et al. Safety of intrauterine devices in MRI. PLoS One 2018;13(10).

21. Committee on Obstetric Practice. Committee Opinion No. 723: guidelines for diagnostic imaging during pregnancy and lactation. Obstet Gynecol 2017;130(4):e210–6.

22. Expert Panel on MRS, Kanal E, Barkovich AJ, et al. ACR guidance document on MR safe practices: 2013. J Magn Reson Imaging 2013;37(3):501–30.

23. Hepper PG, Shahidullah BS. Development of fetal hearing. Arch Dis Child Fetal Neonatal Ed 1994;71(2):F81–7.

24. Hoff MN, McKinney At, Shellock FG, et al. Safety considerations of 7-T MRI in clinical practice. Radiology 2019;292(3):509–18.

25. Glover P, Hykin J, Gowland P, et al. An assessment of the intrauterine sound intensity level during obstetric echo-planar magnetic resonance imaging. Br J Radiol 1995;68(814):1090–4.

26. Richards DS, Frentzen B, Gerhardt KJ, et al. Sound levels in the human uterus. Obstet Gynecol 1992;80(2):186–90.

27. Tirada N, Dreizin D, Khati NJ, et al. Imaging pregnant and lactating patients. Radiographics 2015;35(6):1751–65.

28. Reeves MJ, Brandreth M, Whitby EH, et al. Neonatal cochlear function: measurement after exposure to acoustic noise during in utero MR imaging. Radiology 2010;257(3):802–9.

29. Strizek B, Jani JC, Mucyo E, et al. Safety of MR imaging at 1.5 T in fetuses: a retrospective case-control study of birth weights and the effects of acoustic noise. Radiology 2015;275(2):530–7.

30. Jaimes C, Delgado J, Cunnane MB, et al. Does 3-T fetal MRI induce adverse acoustic effects in the neonate? A preliminary study comparing postnatal auditory test performance of fetuses scanned at 1.5 and 3 T. Pediatr Radiol 2019;49(1):37–45.

31. Kanal E. Gadolinium based contrast agents (GBCA): safety overview after 3 decades of clinical experience. Magn Reson Imaging 2016;34(10):1341–5.

32. Millischer AE, Deloison B, Silvera S, et al. Dynamic contrast enhanced MRI of the placenta: a tool for prenatal diagnosis of placenta accreta? Placenta 2017;53:40–7.

33. Millischer AE, Salomon LJ, Porcher R, et al. Magnetic resonance imaging for abnormally invasive placenta: the added value of intravenous gadolinium injection. BJOG 2017;124(1):88–95.

34. Palacios Jaraquemada JM, Bruno C. Gadolinium-enhanced MR imaging in the differential diagnosis of placenta accreta and placenta percreta. Radiology 2000;216(2):610–1.

35. Tanaka YO, Sohda S, Shigemitsu S, et al. High temporal resolution dynamic contrast MRI in a high risk group for placenta accreta. Magn Reson Imaging 2001;19(5):635–42.

36. Herrey AS, Francis JM, Hughes M, et al. Cardiovascular magnetic resonance can be undertaken in pregnancy and guide clinical decision-making in this patient population. Eur Heart J Cardiovasc Imaging 2019;20(3):291–7.

37. Sikka A, Bisla JK, Rajan PV, et al. How to manage allergic reactions to contrast agent in pregnant patients. AJR Am J Roentgenol 2016;206(2):247–52.

38. Simons FE, Schatz M. Anaphylaxis during pregnancy. J Allergy Clin Immunol 2012;130(3):597–606.

39. Vanden Hoek TL, Morrison LJ, Shuster M, et al. Part 12: cardiac arrest in special situations: 2010

American Heart Association guidelines for cardio-pulmonary resuscitation and emergency cardiovascular care. Circulation 2010;122(18 Suppl 3): S829–61.

40. Horowitz JM, Bisla JK, Yaghmai V. Premedication of pregnant patients with history of iodinated contrast allergy. Abdom Radiol (NY) 2016; 41(12):2424–8.

41. Cowper SE, Robin HS, Steinberg SM, et al. Sclero-myxoedema-like cutaneous diseases in renal-dialysis patients. Lancet 2000;356(9234):1000–1.

42. Grobner T. Gadolinium–a specific trigger for the development of nephrogenic fibrosing dermopathy and nephrogenic systemic fibrosis? Nephrol Dial Transplant 2006;21(4):1104–8.

43. Kaewlai R, Abujudeh H. Nephrogenic systemic fibrosis. AJR Am J Roentgenol 2012;199(1):W17–23.

44. Kanda T, Ishii K, Kawaguchi H, et al. High signal intensity in the dentate nucleus and globus pallidus on unenhanced T1-weighted MR images: relationship with increasing cumulative dose of a gadolinium-based contrast material. Radiology 2014;270(3): 834–41.

45. McDonald RJ, McDonald JS, Kallmes DF, et al. Intra-cranial gadolinium deposition after contrast-enhanced MR imaging. Radiology 2015;275(3): 772–82.

46. De Santis M, Straface G, Cavaliere AF, et al. Gado-linium periconceptional exposure: pregnancy and neonatal outcome. Acta Obstet Gynecol Scand 2007;86(1):99–101.

47. Gibby WA, Gibby KA, Gibby WA. Comparison of Gd DTPA-BMA (Omniscan) versus Gd HP-DO3A (Pro-Hance) retention in human bone tissue by inductively coupled plasma atomic emission spectroscopy. Invest Radiol 2004;39(3):138–42.

48. Murata N, Gonzalez-Cuyar LF, Murata K, et al. Macrocyclic and other non-group 1 gadolinium contrast agents deposit low levels of gadolinium in brain and bone tissue: preliminary results from 9 patients with normal renal function. Invest Radiol 2016; 51(7):447–53.

49. Roberts DR, Lindhorst SM, Welsh CT, et al. High levels of gadolinium deposition in the skin of a patient with normal renal function. Invest Radiol 2016; 51(5):280–9.

50. White GW, Gibby WA, Tweedle MF. Comparison of Gd(DTPA-BMA) (Omniscan) versus Gd(HP-DO3A) (ProHance) relative to gadolinium retention in human bone tissue by inductively coupled plasma mass spectroscopy. Invest Radiol 2006;41(3):272–8.

51. Fraum TJ, Ludwig DR, Bashir MR, et al. Gadolinium-based contrast agents: a comprehensive risk assessment. J Magn Reson Imaging 2017;46(2): 338–53.

52. Puac P, Rodriguez A, Vallejo C, et al. Safety of contrast material use during pregnancy and lactation. Magn Reson Imaging Clin N Am 2017; 25(4):787–97.

53. Novak Z, Thurmond AS, Ross PL, et al. Gadolinium-DTPA transplacental transfer and distribution in fetal tissue in rabbits. Invest Radiol 1993;28(9):828–30.

54. Tremblay E, Therasse E, Thomassin-Naggara I, et al. Quality initiatives: guidelines for use of medical imaging during pregnancy and lactation. Radio-graphics 2012;32(3):897–911.

55. Oh KY, Roberts VH, Schabel MC, et al. Gadolinium chelate contrast material in pregnancy: fetal bio-distribution in the nonhuman primate. Radiology 2015;276(1):110–8.

56. Jain C. ACOG Committee opinion no. 723: guide-lines for diagnostic imaging during pregnancy and lactation. Obstet Gynecol 2019;133(1):186.

57. Bashir MR, Bhatti L, Marin D, et al. Emerging applications for ferumoxytol as a contrast agent in MRI. J Magn Reson Imaging 2015;41(4):884–98.

58. Vasanawala SS, Nguyen KL, Hope MD, et al. Safety and technique of ferumoxytol administration for MRI. Magn Reson Med 2016;75(5):2107–11.

59. Pai AB, Garba AO. Ferumoxytol: a silver lining in the treatment of anemia of chronic kidney disease or another dark cloud? J Blood Med 2012;3:77–85.

60. Bailie GR. Adverse events associated with intrave-nous iron preparations: a comparison of reported rates. Clin Adv Hematol Oncol 2012;10(9):600–2.

61. Santosh S, Podaralla P, Miller B. Anaphylaxis with elevated serum tryptase after administration of intra-venous ferumoxytol. NDT Plus 2010;3(4):341–2.

62. Storey P, Lim RP, Chandarana H, et al. MRI assess-ment of hepatic iron clearance rates after USPIO administration in healthy adults. Invest Radiol 2012;47(12):717–24.

63. FDA. Full prescribing information: feraheme. Avail-able at: https://www.accessdata.fda.gov/drugsatfda_docs/label/2018/022180s009lbl.pdf. Accessed January 31, 2020.

64. Myllynen PK, Loughran MJ, Howard CV, et al. Ki-netics of gold nanoparticles in the human placenta. Reprod Toxicol 2008;26(2):130–7.

65. Zhu A, Reeder SB, Johnson KM, et al. Quantitative ferumoxytol-enhanced MRI in pregnancy: a feasi-bility study in the nonhuman primate. Magn Reson Imaging 2020;65:100–8.

66. Bird ST, Gelperin K, Sahin L, et al. First-trimester exposure to gadolinium-based contrast agents: a utilization study of 4.6 million U.S. pregnancies. Radiology 2019;293(1):193–200.

67. Kallmes DF, Watson RE Jr. Gadolinium administra-tion in undetected pregnancy: cause for alarm? Radiology 2019;293(1):201–2.

68. Baheti AD, Nicola R, Bennett GL, et al. Magnetic resonance imaging of abdominal and pelvic pain in the pregnant patient. Magn Reson Imaging Clin N Am 2016;24(2):403–17.

69. Sachs HC, Committee On D. The transfer of drugs and therapeutics into human breast milk: an update on selected topics. Pediatrics 2013;132(3): e796–809.

70. Han F, Rapacchi S, Khan S, et al. Four-dimensional, multiphase, steady-state imaging with contrast enhancement (MUSIC) in the heart: a feasibility study in children. Magn Reson Med 2015;74(4): 1042–9.

71. Lai LM, Cheng JY, Alley MT, et al. Feasibility of ferumoxytol-enhanced neonatal and young infant cardiac MRI without general anesthesia. J Magn Reson Imaging 2017;45(5):1407–18.

72. Ning P, Zucker EJ, Wong P, et al. Hemodynamic safety and efficacy of ferumoxytol as an intravenous contrast agents in pediatric patients and young adults. Magn Reson Imaging 2016;34(2): 152–8.

73. Ruangwattanapaisarn N, Hsiao A, Vasanawala SS. Ferumoxytol as an off-label contrast agent in body 3T MR angiography: a pilot study in children. Pediatr Radiol 2015;45(6):831–9.

The Physics of Magnetic Resonance Imaging Safety

Roger Jason Stafford, PhD

KEYWORDS

- Magnetic resonance safety • Static magnetic field • Spatial field gradient
- Pulsed gradient magnetic field • Radiofrequency field • Heating • Acoustic noise
- Peripheral stimulation

KEY POINTS

- The primary safety risks in MRI arise from the 3 unique magnetic fields used: the static magnetic field (B0), the time-varying radiofrequency magnetic field (B1) and the time-varying gradient magnetic field (dB/dt). Understanding and controlling the spatiotemporal distribution of these fields helps ensure MR safety for patients.
- Static magnetic field risk is dominated by the potential for ferromagnetic objects brought into the room to become projectiles as well as potential displacement, disruption, or damage to external or implanted devices.
- Diffuse heating from the time-varying radiofrequency magnetic field is characterized by the specific absorption rate to help manage core body temperature and avoid undue thermal stress on patients.
- Focal heating from the time-varying radiofrequency magnetic field can arise from interaction with conducting materials in the bore and is one of the most often reported injuries. Minimizing conductors in the bore, avoiding close proximity of conductors to each other, and insulation between patient and conducting surfaces can help mitigate risks.
- The time-varying gradient magnetic field can induce peripheral nerve stimulation in patients and is also the source of acoustic noise requiring hearing protection in MRI. This field can also interact with external or implanted medical devices as well, possibly resulting in unintended stimulation, as well as disruption or damage of the implant.

INTRODUCTION

Compared with other advanced tomographic imaging modalities, magnetic resonance (MR) imaging is an extremely versatile modality capable of exquisite soft tissue contrast as well as functional and metabolic information. As technology has advanced, costs for high-performance systems have come down, and wider availability and clinical acceptance of this modality have grown, so have use and demand. MR imaging is now ubiquitous in radiology departments worldwide and is rapidly expanding to areas outside traditional diagnostic radiology departments, such as interventional, intraoperative, or radiation oncology hybrid suites.

MR imaging is a nonionizing radiation modality. The safety considerations and risks are unique and radically different from routine imaging sources using ionizing radiation. In the hands of, or under the direct supervision of, properly trained personnel, MR imaging is one of the safest imaging modalities. However, because of the propensity for serious or life-threatening injury to untrained personnel even entering the MR environment, a highly structured set of safety guidelines are used to help minimize the risk associated with MR imaging.[1,2]

Department of Imaging Physics, The University of Texas MD Anderson Cancer Center, 1400 Pressler Street, Unit 1472, Houston, TX 77030, USA
E-mail address: jstafford@mdanderson.org

Magn Reson Imaging Clin N Am 28 (2020) 517–536
https://doi.org/10.1016/j.mric.2020.08.002
1064-9689/20/© 2020 Elsevier Inc. All rights reserved.

The Earth's magnetic field is on the order of 0.5 G (0.05 mT, where 1 T = 10,000 G). The unique safety concerns in MR imaging are caused by the generation and/or presence of 3 independent magnetic fields used for imaging by the MR scanner:

- Static magnetic field (B_0): a very strong magnetic field (0.5–7 T) is used to generate a potential energy difference in tissue proton spin population. This field, and the large spatial field gradients (T/m) associated with sharp transitions near the scanner, are the source for potentially large magnetic forces on objects entering the MR environment and can also potentially affect devices and personnel outside the MR suite. For most scanners in use today, this field is usually generated by large currents circulating in cryogen-cooled superconducting coils and so are generally always on, making the safety concerns caused by this field omnipresent and requiring substantial access and supervisory control and vigilance over personnel and items entering the MR environment.
- Time-varying radiofrequency (RF) magnetic field (B_1): a much smaller magnetic field (μT) oscillating at or near the MR frequency (megahertz) of protons is generated orthogonal to the static field by another set of current-carrying coils close to the patient but inside the bore of the MR scanner during imaging to excite and/or manipulate the polarized spins for signal and contrast. This field, characterized by its amplitude, frequency, and duty cycle, is responsible for risks caused by heating in the bore of the scanner. This field is only on during imaging.
- Time-varying magnetic field gradient (G): 3 orthogonal linear gradient magnetic fields (mT/m) are generated by another set of coils in the bore and are pulsed for image encoding and contrast manipulation during image acquisition. This rapid switching of the large currents through these coils is the generating source of the loud acoustic noise generated during MR imaging, whereas the rapid switching of the resulting magnetic field (dB/dt) at points in the gradient field can cause muscle stimulation.

Magnetic Resonance Safety Operating Modes

The output of these fields on the scanner is tightly controlled. In the United States, the Food and Drug Administration (FDA) provides guidelines for marketing of clinical MR scanners. Most safety limits and nomenclature used by the FDA come from the International Electrotechnical Commission (IEC) publication 60601-2-33, "Requirements for the Safety of MR Equipment for Medical Diagnosis." These agencies have established different operating modes for MR imaging based on the exposure of the patient to each of the 3 magnetic fields and the likelihood that this exposure may cause stress to the patient. Normal operating mode is one in which there is no expectation that scanning will result in physiologic stress and can be used safely for all patients. First-level controlled operating mode is one in which 1 or more outputs may reach a value that may cause physiologic stress to patients. It is expected that this mode is used to achieve a clinical benefit to the patient that outweighs these risks and that appropriate medical supervision is provided. There is a second-level controlled mode that allows higher outputs that can be used for research purposes after review by an independent review board for ethical and safety consideration.

Note that MR scanner operating modes govern outputs designed to manage physiologic stress to the patient and do not relate directly to prevention of safety events associated with improper patient screening or positioning as well as devices in the MR environment. These events are prevented by learning and understanding the appropriate use of the equipment. Similarly, although operating modes and associated outputs are often cited as part of the technical conditions for safely scanning medical implants, these modes and output measures were not created with those objectives in mind, but they are often the only way of specifying system output in a way that the user has control over.

There are many excellent reviews on the MR physics underlying MR safety.[3–7] This article reviews some of the practical aspects of physics needed to understand the system operation, outputs, and basic interactions with tissue and other materials with a view to underscoring how this information may be translated into the clinical management of patients or operation of the scanner.

STATIC MAGNETIC FIELD

The primary safety concerns to consider with a strong static magnetic field include potential direct interaction with patient (biological effects); ferromagnetic objects becoming projectiles (missile effect); interference or damage of ancillary medical equipment; disruption, damage, or displacement of implanted medical devices; and, for superconducting systems, cryogen safety considerations.

A strong, static magnetic field is used to polarize the spins. The field acts as a reservoir of potential energy for the spins. The stronger the static magnetic field, the larger population of spins aligned with the field and hence the larger potential signal that can be produced by the system. Large magnetic field strengths are typically cited in Tesla (T), whereas smaller fields, such as the so-called fringe fields further from the magnet, may be cited in Gauss (1 G = 0.1 mT). Current clinical imaging field strength ranges from 0.2 T to 7.0 T, with most current systems being 1.5-T or 3.0-T fields generated by cylindrical superconducting magnet technology. These field strengths are on the order of 50,000 times the Earth's magnetic field. Of course, objects exposed to these fields can be subject to varying degrees of magnetic force.

For siting purposes, magnets used for MR imaging tend to have a very high, homogeneous static magnetic field over a spherical volume for imaging (ie, 50 × 50 × 50 cm), and then have a very sharp spatial field gradient moving away from the imaging volume to minimize the penetration of the fringe magnetic field into the surrounding area and help keep within a controlled area, such as the MR suite.

Magnetic fields are generated by charges in motion (ie, currents) and it is often convenient to represent this source current density in terms of a magnetic dipole moment, which is a measure of the potential interaction between this current density and an externally applied magnetic field.

Magnetic Materials

Magnetic materials are those in which an applied external magnetic field can induce a net magnetization (M) from the current density induced within the material.[8] The ratio of magnetization induced per unit magnetic field strength is called the magnetic susceptibility (χ) and is a property of the material. Although the relationship can be complicated for three-dimensional materials, generally the induced magnetization is proportional to the local magnetic flux density (B), with the proportionality constant being a function of the susceptibility.

Most materials encountered in routine clinical imaging lie in the range of approximately $-10^{-5} < \chi < 10^{-5}$. Diamagnetic materials (ie, water, soft tissue, deoxygenated blood, copper) generally resist the applied field and hence have a small induced magnetism against the field ($-10^{-5} < \chi < 0$). Paramagnetic materials (ie, gadolinium, calcium, titanium) have a weak induced magnetism that aligns with the applied field ($0 < \chi < 10^{-5}$). Water

susceptibility is approximately -9×10^{-6} and susceptibility differences greater than 10^{-5} from this value are likely to result in substantial artifacts and distortion on MR images.

In the paramagnetic and diamagnetic materials described earlier, generally no appreciable forces are observed on these objects at current field strengths used in MR imaging. However, ferromagnetic materials (ie, iron, stainless steels, cobalt, nickel) have unique magnetic domains that result in a much stronger induced magnetization from susceptibility ($\chi > 10^{-2}$). Therefore, in addition to substantial artifacts and distortion that may negate the diagnostic quality of the acquired images, much stronger magnetic forces exist on these materials when placed in an external magnetic field. The forces on these objects are a paramount safety concern.

Forces on Magnetic Materials

Of the magnetic materials discussed, it is ferromagnetic objects that experience the greatest forces in the MR environment. The external static magnetic field induces a field in the object as characterized by its large susceptibility. However, these materials generally can only be magnetized up to a point before reaching a maximal saturating magnetization (M_s). Typically, ferromagnetic objects saturate between 0.25 and 2.5 T, depending on the material, with iron at the highest end of the scale. In addition to size and shape, this can affect the net induced magnetization. The external field can result in a demagnetization factor such that the magnetic susceptibility becomes a strong function of object shape, which can be characterized by a shape-dependent susceptibility constant, χ_D,[8,9] which accounts for this demagnetization effect.

The net induced magnetization in magnetic objects creates an effective net dipole moment (m) in the material. The potential energy (U) between this dipole moment and the external field is given by $U = - m \bullet B$. This dot product shows that the energy of the system depends on both the magnitude of these values and their alignment with each other. Energy is minimized with the dipole moments and field aligned with each other. Forces arise on objects in a potential field when there are spatial gradients in the field. In general, $F = \nabla U$. This treatment shows 2 primary forces of concern for objects placed in a magnetic field: displacement forces arising from spatial variations in the magnetic field itself, and rotational forces (torques) attempting to align the dipole moment with the external magnetic field.

Magnetically Induced Displacement Force

Strong displacement forces on a magnetic material arise from the spatial variations (gradients) in the static magnetic field (*B*). The relationship between the displacement force (F_d) experienced by a magnetic object with a dipole moment (*m*) object in a static magnetic field (*B*) can be represented by the relationship:[9]

$$F_d \propto |\nabla(m \cdot B)| \propto V \cdot M |\nabla B| \qquad \textbf{Equation 1}$$

That is, the force on the object is strongly dependent on the mass of magnetic material, via the volume (*V*), the induced magnetization (*M*) in the magnetic material from its susceptibility (χ) and static magnetic field value at a particular location, and the spatial gradient of the static magnetic field ($|\nabla B|$) at that location. So, for objects in an appreciable magnetic field, force increases where rapid changes in the magnetic field (ie, high spatial field gradients) exist. These areas are conspicuous on isofield plots provided by the vendor because these are usually represented by tighter clusters of field lines. Objects are likely to accelerate their greatest in these regions. For a cylindrical-bore, superconducting-magnet design, these gradients are greatest at the magnet face and the edges of the bore (**Fig. 1**).

An obvious reference force for displacement is the weight of the object from gravity (F_g). As F_d becomes appreciable, the object may move on smooth surfaces on which there is little or no opposing frictional force. However, as the force of gravity is exceeded, unrestrained objects may begin to levitate and accelerate into the magnet bore. In particular, ferromagnetic objects may accelerate with a force many times their weight. To get an understanding of these values, the ratio of these forces can be approximated by:

$$\frac{F_d}{F_g} \cong C \cdot M \cdot |\nabla B| \qquad \textbf{Equation 2}$$

where the constant of proportionality is related to the object density (ρ), permeability of free space (μ_0), and gravitational constant via $C = (\rho\,\mu_0\,g)^{-1}$. Note, as discussed previously, the amount of magnetization that can be induced in a ferromagnetic object is limited ($M \leq M_s$) and so an object placed in the static magnetic field does not necessarily yield an induced magnetism $M = B$ in regions of higher magnetic inductance, but tracks with the local value of *B* until reaching M_s.

By way of example, for fully saturated iron, $M \sim 2.2$ T and $C \sim 10$ ($\rho = 7900$ kg/m^3; $\mu_0 = 4\pi \times 10^{-7}$ H/m, and $g = 9.8$ m/s^2). Just inside and near the edge of the bore of a 3-T scanner, the spatial field gradient can exceed 5 T/m, resulting in forces exceeding 120 times the weight of the object. However, the trouble with controlling object displacements starts much further away than that. At 0.4 to 0.5 m from the bore face, where the object is not fully saturated and the field is less than one-tenth of its maximum, the displacement force may still be strong enough to exceed the weight of the object, depending on the size and magnetization properties of the material. Going out to the edge of the patient table, where the field can be in the range of 3 to 5 mT, forces can still be appreciable enough to move unrestrained or unhindered objects.[10]

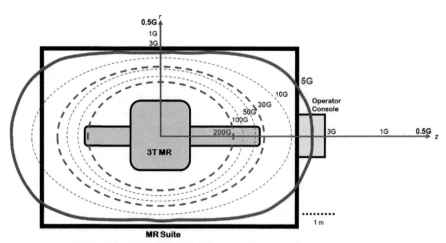

Fig. 1. Fringe field of a typical MR imaging suite showing the 5-G limit. All areas containing the 5-G line, including above and below the unit, must be access controlled. Because this safety limit is attributed to medical implants (eg, pacemakers), screening of personnel is required before entering. The 30-G zone is the limit for significant kinetic forces to be exerted on ferromagnetic objects. Refer to **Table 1** for a summary of relevant isofield regions and distances from the magnet. Units: 1 G = 0.1 mT.

Of course, for medical implants that may enter the MR imaging scanner, it is important to assess the magnitude of the displacement force on the object. To this end, a simple deflection test has been devised in which the object is suspended and a protractor used to measure the maximal potential displacement location of the object, which is where the maximal spatial field gradient occurs near the edge of the face of the magnet. The angle of deflection can be compared against the force of gravity on the object, with a 45° deflection being the point at which $F_d/F_g \geq 1$. From this information, maximal static field and spatial field gradient conditions can be elucidated.[11–14]

Displacement forces are therefore the first forces experienced as objects or people enter the MR environment. As shown later, forces that may affect implanted medical devices can extend outside the room containing the scanner. Given the acute nature of the problem, safety interlocks by way of access control and screening of both objects and personnel have been put in place to reduce the risks associated with the MR environment. Note that the location and magnitude of these forces depend on both the value and spatial gradient of the static magnetic field in a given location. These properties vary as a function of magnet design characteristics, such as field strength, active versus passive shielding, and bore dimensions. Knowledge of the areas where the forces are significant and for what objects is necessary for maintaining a safe environment and is needed for each installation. Plots of the magnetic field, spatial field gradient, and product of magnetic field and spatial field gradient is one way of obtaining this information, and some form of this information is supplied by the vendor operator manuals for safety considerations.[10,15]

Magnetically Induced Torque

In asymmetric magnetic objects (ie, ellipsoidal or elongated), a strong net dipole moment not aligned with the static magnetic field may be present. In order to achieve the lowest energy state, a rotational force (torque) attempts to align the dipole with the external field. The torque (**L**) generated by this force is proportional to the cross-product between the dipole moment (**m**) and magnetic field (**B**).[3,4,9]

$$L \propto m \times B \Rightarrow L \propto V \cdot M \cdot B \cdot sin\theta \quad \textbf{Equation 3}$$

Similar to the displacement force, the total torque depends on the amount of the magnetized material (V) and induced magnetization (M); however, it also depends directly on field strength (B)

and not the spatial gradient, as well as the angle between **m** and **B** (θ). This equation indicates that, if the dipole of the object manages to align itself with the field, the torque goes away. The maximum torque experienced by the object can be represented by the following relation:

$$L_{max} \propto V \cdot M_s^2 \cdot \chi_D^2 \quad \textbf{Equation 4}$$

For ferromagnetic objects subject to demagnetization factors, it can be seen that, as the field increased, the dependence of the torque becomes a function of the object size, the saturated magnetization of the object, and a strongly shape-dependent modified susceptibility coefficient that accounts for the demagnetization effects.[16] In general, elongated objects experience the strongest torques, whereas more isotropic objects experience less.

Obviously, a torque on an implanted device in a patient can cause harm if strong enough to break free. Measurement of magnetically induced torque on a ferromagnetic device or implant can be performed by affixing the object in a rigid holder attached to a torsion spring and measuring the maximum deflection.[16] Similar to the deflection comparison with the force from the object weight, if the measured torque is less than the length of the object times the force of gravity, the object is unlikely to carry significant additional risk. These thresholds are both conservative and may not prohibit entry into the MR environment depending on how the device is secured in place. This test is often coupled with the deflection test for displacement force[11] to assess risk of an object in the bore of the magnet. For larger objects for which these tests are either inappropriate or the device is not designed to enter the bore, customized tests may need to be performed to establish some reasonable set of conditions for safe use of the equipment in the MR environment.[17]

Note that a weaker torque may be experienced by conducting objects moving within the magnetic field. As mentioned earlier, when magnetic flux through a conducting object, such as from motion, is changing, Faraday's law indicates that eddy currents arise in the object in proportion to the rate of change of flux. Lenz's law further states that this force works to oppose the motion generating force. This force on conductors can result in some unexpected dampening or resistance of large conductors to motion in the magnet. For nonferrous objects, such as metal heart valves, moving rapidly in the magnetic field, it raises concerns that this force may be substantial enough to hinder normal valve function and require additional monitoring of the patient during MR imaging, particularly as higher magnetic fields are used for imaging.[18,19]

Cryogen Concerns

An additional safety concern with superconducting magnets is the substantial amount of liquid helium used to supercool the coils. If a leak develops, the helium can enter the room as a colorless and odorless gas that displaces oxygen and may result in asphyxiation. The Occupational Safety and Health Administration (OSHA) standard states that oxygen depletion in an enclosed space resulting in less than 19.5% oxygen is hazardous to unprotected personnel (29 CFR 1910.146). In addition, MR systems are at risk of a quench. A quench is a sudden loss in the superconductivity of the magnet when the cryogen cooling is no longer sufficient to maintain this state. The time for a typical 1.5-T to 3.0-T magnet to go from field to 20 to 50 mT is on the order of 20 to 120 seconds (depending on the magnet design and field strength). Loss of superconductivity means a high resistance is suddenly present in the coils and the several hundred Amperes of current quickly generates substantial heating. Heating of the liquid helium causes it to boil off as an extremely cold gas. The liquid to gas transition results in a tremendous volume expansion. Gas is expelled from the room to the outside via a quench pipe. If the quench pipe fails, wholly or in part, the cold helium gas will enter the examination room and may result in hypothermia or asphyxiation. Emergency procedures for addressing a quench incident should be developed for all MR imaging facilities, but, importantly, should also be initially addressed during facility siting and design.

Static Magnetic Field Safety Limits

The magnetic forces in MR imaging do interact with human physiology.[20] Possible side effects of moving or working in higher fields (ie, ≥ 2 T) include transient nausea, vertigo, metallic taste, and/or phosphenes.[20,21] Effects can be minimized by moving slower (ie, ≤ 3 T/s)[10] when near the front of the bore and have not proved to be of significant concern at field strengths up to 3 T.[22] Magnetohydrodynamic effects on flowing blood can result in increased T waves on electrocardiogram (ECG), which can lead to issues with both proper monitoring of patients and triggering acquisitions.[23] Although systems with higher field strengths are entering the market, the FDA has noted that patient exposure to static magnetic fields less than or equal to 8 T for adults, children, and infants more than 1 month of age is not considered a significant risk.[24]

Electronically powered or magnetically programmed active implanted medical devices (AIMDs), include device families such as cardiac implanted electronic devices (CIEDs), brain/nerve/spine/bladder stimulators, and drug infusion pumps. AIMDs may not only suffer from issues of displacement forces or torques as passive devices do but may also be susceptible to temporary or permanent B_0-field–induced device malfunction.[25] One prominent example of this type of disruption is that of the impact of the magnetic field on the reed switch of CIED. The reed switch enables an external magnet to be used to program the pacing or therapy delivery mode of the device. Exposure to the MR environment without disabling this switch in older non-MR conditional CIEDs, and appropriately monitoring the patient, has resulted in fatality.[26] Because of the sensitivity of such devices, any area containing fringe static magnetic fields of 0.5 mT (5 G) or higher must be controlled and clearly marked,[15,25] with personnel being screened for these and other implanted devices before entry.[1,2] Note that this controlled zone can extend above or below the MR suite as well as around.

Static Magnetic Field Safety Summary

Magnetic field bioeffects do not present a high-risk safety issue at routine clinical field strengths (≤ 3 T). However, the potential for ferromagnetic objects to be pulled violently into the magnet (missile effect) is the primary safety risk from the static magnetic field and is second to RF-induced thermal injury in terms of reported safety events related to MR system magnetic fields.[27] The forces on these large, heavy objects are high enough to result in severe injury or death to anyone caught between the object and its path to the magnet, and the difference between a moderate pull on the object and substantial forces is just a few meters (see Fig. 1). Similarly, the static magnetic field may present a hazard to patients with ferromagnetic implants because of strong displacement forces, which are maximal as the patient passes the mouth of the bore because of the high spatial field gradients (Fig. 2), as well as strong torques, which are maximal in the region around magnet isocenter (Table 1).

These strong fields can also damage and disrupt normal operation of AIMDs, such as pacemakers, at a distance far from the magnet isocenter in the fringe fields. For this reason, access to areas containing this region must be identified and tightly access controlled. Note that, during initial siting or site safety reviews, these fields extend above and below the magnet as well as all around the

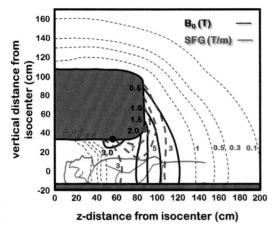

Fig. 2. The approximate location and magnitude of B_0 isofield lines (*black*) in units of Tesla and spatial field gradient (SFG) lines (*red*) in units of T/m as a patient enters a 3 T scanner. The maximum field (*black circle*) is within the bore and is approximately 3.5 T, whereas the maximum SFG (*red circle*) is located at the bore opening and is approximately 10 T/m. The region of extremely high spatial gradient–generated displacement force that may be a hazard to patients with ferromagnetic medical implants is emphasized with bold SFG lines (>3 T/m) and begins at the bore opening. Further inside the bore, magnetic torque forces become stronger and are the dominant consideration as the spatial gradients weaken near magnet isocenter. Vendors often quote the maximum SFG exposure within a cylindrical region so that users can understand the maximum SFG that might be experienced by a particular device or implant on the patient. Units: 1 T/m = 100 G/cm.

system and may penetrate into adjacent spaces and present a safety hazard or affect nearby sensitive equipment (see **Table 1**). Note that a magnet located on an upper floor with fringe field lines going out the window still may present a hazard to the window washers or the equipment they use. It is important to fully assess the location and potential impacts of the magnet fringe fields. Modern scanners actively shield their systems to minimize the range of this field. In some cases, permeable metal magnetic shielding may be needed to confine the fringe fields to the MR suite.

In addition, the cryogens associated with cooling the superconducting coils needed to generate the static magnetic field are a safety concern as well. Helium leaks can displace the oxygen in the room, resulting in risk of asphyxiation. Accidental or controlled magnet quenches run a risk of a violent release of helium gas into the MR room, or exposure of personnel at the output of the quench pipe. Quench procedures tailored to the specific facility and routine checking of the quench pipe are needed.

TIME-VARYING RADIOFREQUENCY MAGNETIC FIELD

Polarized spins aligned with the static magnetic field are modulated using RF magnetic field pulses tuned to or near the resonant (Larmor) frequency for both signal generation and contrast manipulation purposes. The resonance frequency is the product of the gyromagnetic ratio (γ) of the imaged nuclei and the static field strength (B_0). For protons, γ = 42.58 MHz/T, yielding resonance frequencies (*f*) of approximately 64 MHz and 128 MHz for 1.5 T and 3.0 T respectively. At these frequencies, the primary safety concerns are whole-body and localized heating from the absorption of the applied RF energy.[28] Understanding and controlling this heating is paramount in MR imaging because thermal injury is the most prevalent reported injury.[27]

A fraction of the energy in the applied RF magnetic field (B_1) is absorbed, resulting in heating. From Maxwell's equations, a time-varying B_1 field is the source of an induced electric field (E_1), from which a current density (J_C) is generated via tissue conductivity (σ). Simultaneously, the time rate of change of this induced E_1 field gives rise to an opposing displacement current (J_D) via the tissue permittivity (ε). The total induced current (J) would then be given by the expression in Equation 5 as:

$$J = J_C + J_D = \sigma E_1 + \varepsilon \frac{\partial E_1}{\partial t} \qquad \textbf{Equation 5}$$

Thus, the dielectric properties of the medium determine conversion of the applied RF field to currents that are ultimately absorbed locally, resulting in tissue heating. Because this is the key means of heating, at the wavelength used in MR imaging, a large fraction of the energy is deposited superficially, with less heating observed at depth.

The amplitude (B_{1p}) of the applied RF magnetic field used in MR imaging is much smaller (μT) than either the static or gradient magnetic fields and is applied on the order of milliseconds using high-power (kilowatt) amplifiers to drive whole-body or head/extremity-sized multirung, circularly polarized transmit coils. Remembering that the spins are polarized to have a net magnetization aligned with the direction of B_0, the applied B_1 field is often designated by a superscript (B_1^+), which signifies the excitation pulse is circularly polarized along this direction. Polarization of the excitation pulse has an efficiency advantage in that the applied power is primarily used to excite the spins polarized with the field magnetic field, as opposed to linear polarization, which wastefully excites both B_1^+ and B_1^-

Table 1
Summary of general static field regions, limits, and potential hazards in a magnetic resonance imaging suite with sample approximate distances for an actively shielded, wide-bore 3-T scanner

Field Strength	Location	Significance and Potential Disruptive Impact
0.05 mT (0.5 G)	r = 3.5 m z = 8.5 m	Earth's magnetic field (average)
0.05–3 mT (0.5–30 G)	r = 3.5–2.0 m z = 8.5–3.0 m	Medical equipment: photomultiplier tubes, image intensifiers, gamma cameras, PET, cyclotrons, electron microscopes, linear accelerators, ultrasonography, x-ray tubes, computed tomography units, color/monochrome monitors AIMDs: CIED, stimulators, insulin pumps, hearing implants Devices: watches, small motors, cameras, credit cards, magnetic data carriers, processors, oscilloscopes
0.5 mT (5 G)	r = 2.5 m z = 4.5 m	**Controlled access to MR environment limit** **Mandatory posting of potential safety hazards** **Mandatory personnel screening**
3 mT (30 G)	r = 2.0 m z = 3.0 m	Threshold for onset of kinetic energy hazards from small ferrous objects
20 mT (200 G)	r = 1.75 m z = 2.3 m	**Often used as limit for movement of ferrous objects within room (ie, for service personnel)**
20–500 mT (200–5000 G)	$r \leq$ 1.75 m z = 2.3–1.3 m	Range of MR conditional anesthesia, patient monitoring, injectors location/tethering limits
High SFG (≥3 T/m)	Bore entry z = 1.1–0.7 m	**Region of strongest magnetic displacement forces** **Largest risk for ferromagnetic implants**
1.5–3.0 T	Isocenter	Region of strongest magnetic torque forces Field strengths for most commercial MR imaging
>3.0 T	Isocenter	First level controlled operating mode for B_0
7 T	Isocenter	Current highest commercial field strength
>8.0 T	Isocenter	Second level controlled operating mode

See **Figs. 1** and **2** for visualization of regions.

precessing spins. The B_{1p} for a rectangular pulse is approximated by $\alpha/\gamma\tau_{rf}$, where α is the flip angle and τ_{rf} is the time the pulse is played out (ie, inverse of bandwidth). Note the lack of dependence on the value of B_0. This calculation yields 11.7 μT for a 1-millisecond 180° pulse. Many RF pulses are optimized (ie, timing, spatial-spectral selectivity, power, and so forth) and so do not have such a simple dependence on these parameters, but the case discussed earlier is illustrative nonetheless.

The B_1^+ field has wavelength $\lambda = c/f$, where c is the speed of light (3 × 10^8 m/s), which is about 4.7 m and 2.3 m for 1.5 T and 3.0 T respectively. However, of interested here is propagation through the body, which has different dielectric properties than air. Assuming a relative permittivity ε_r = 60 (muscle), a new, much smaller wavelength of $\lambda_{tissue} = \lambda_{air}/\sqrt{\varepsilon_r}$ would be expected, which is about 50 cm and 25 cm for 1.5 T and 3.0 T

respectively. So, the effective wavelengths get smaller with increasing field strength and with tissue permittivity. The smaller wavelengths affect patients more strongly, affecting both propagation through the patient as well as absorption of energy.

The power applied to tissue is generally a function of field strength, pulse sequence, and patient size. A fraction is absorbed in patient, implants, and/or conductors as heat. The primary safety concerns are heat stress from sustained whole-body temperature increases and potential for tissue damage from localized high-temperature exposures. Although temperature control is the aim, temperature cannot be easily measured internally during routine clinical MR imaging. So, temperature control in MR imaging focuses on controlling system power output in conjunction with theoretic and/or empirical thresholds of damage.

Specific Absorption Rate

The rate of energy deposition in tissue is the specific absorption rate (SAR), which is often expressed in units of watts per kilogram. Absent any losses, the initial change in temperature (ΔT) in time (Δt) is proportional to the SAR via the heat capacity (C) of the material so that $\Delta T = C \cdot SAR \cdot \Delta t$. Therefore, for an insulated slab with $C = 3.5$ kJ/kg/°C (similar to tissue), this simple estimate with a SAR of 1 W/kg results in a 1°C temperature increase in 1 hour. In 15 minutes, 2 W/kg results in a 0.5°C increase and 4 W/kg results in a 1°C increase.

Ignoring the impact of permittivity in Equation 5, a relationship between the applied B_1^+ peak amplitude (B_p), induced electric field (E_p), and SAR for a homogeneous spherical object of radius (R) and density (ρ) can be approximated by[3,4]

$$SAR = \frac{\sigma |E_p|^2}{2\rho} = \frac{\sigma}{2\rho} \cdot (\pi \cdot R \cdot f \cdot B_p)^2 \cdot D$$

Equation 6

where the tissue conductivity (σ) generally ranges from about 0.4 to 1.0 S/m for soft tissue for the Larmor frequencies ($f = \gamma B_0$) used in clinical MR imaging, with progressively lower values for tissue such as lung, bone, and adipose that are in the range of 0.1 to 0.3 S/m.[29]

The duty cycle (D) is a factor that reduces the SAR based on the ratio of time the RF pulse is on versus the time period over which it is averaged and is determined by the pulse sequence parameters used during imaging. For many two-dimensional acquisitions, the duty cycle can be estimated as $D = (\tau_{rf} \cdot N_{echoes} \cdot N_{slices})/TR$. Here TR is the pulse repetition time (milliseconds), τ_{rf} is the RF pulse duration (milliseconds), with N_{echoes} and N_{slices} being the number of interleaved echoes and/or slices per TR period. Noting that B_p depends on the RF pulse flip angle (α) used, $SAR \sim B_0^2 \cdot \alpha^2 \cdot D$ (patient size). Control over the flip angle and duty cycle are 2 powerful means for controlling SAR from an acquisition standpoint. Some suggestions for reducing SAR in MR scanning are given in **Table 2**.

To illustrate the magnitude of the effect, a simple calculation is instructional using a spin-echo acquisition applied to a spherical object with $R = 10$ cm (ie, human head), $\sigma = 0.5$ S/m, $\rho = 1000$ kg/m^3, and $B_p = 10$ µT for 0.5 millisecond (180° pulse). One 90° to 180° sequence per slice and TR = 400 millisecond, with 15 slices per TR period, gives $D = 0.03$, resulting in an estimated SAR = 0.3 W/kg.

Of course, a more detailed spatiotemporal estimation of SAR in human patients is more complicated and requires realistic modeling of the transmitted RF field propagation, absorption, and bioheat transfer in tissue. A great deal of research has been done in this area and very accurate simulation is possible to aid in characterizing heating, such as for investigating safety issues associated with higher field strengths or medical implants in the MR environment.[30–34]

MR scanners provide a conservative estimate of SAR during prescription of pulse sequences using a process that requires both system-specific and patient-specific information as input. The B_1^+ power needed to excite the spins is estimated via a prescan calibration process and can be used to make SAR predictions. This information is combined with information about the pulses and timing used in the prescribed pulse sequence to estimate $B_1^+{}_{rms}$ for the sequence over an appropriate averaging time, such as the TR period. During the scan, RF power delivered to the patient is estimated in real time using the pulse-energy method[10,35] to update predictions. In either case, the estimated power delivered to the patient is normalized by the patient weight to estimate whole-body SAR. Peak SAR can be roughly estimated to be approximately 2.5 times higher.[36] Partial-body SAR is useful when the amount of tissue exposed is reduced (ie, head transmit coil) and is calculated by estimating the mass for normalization from the fraction of exposed tissue in the coil. Whole-body, partial-body, and head SAR are calculated for volume excitation coils. When local excitation coils are used, whole-body and local SAR, power averaged over any 10 g of the patient's body, are used to control the system output.[37]

Radiofrequency Field Safety Limits

SAR is a measure of RF power absorbed in tissue, and the estimate of this system output operates as a surrogate for managing temperature effects in MR imaging because patient temperature is not easily measured in the area of heating during imaging. Whole-body and localized heating are the primary concerns with absorption of RF power during imaging. The thermoregulatory system helps the body counteract this thermal stress and manages through a combination of heat radiation and evaporation from the surface of the body as well as convection and conduction. For the exposures expected in MR imaging, this means the patient may feel heat sensations in the skin, increased perspiration, and increased pulse rate.

So, with respect to temperature effects, whole-body RF field exposures resulting in less than or

Table 2
Summary of common specific absorption rate reduction techniques for magnetic resonance acquisitions

Acquisition Modification	Potential Tradeoff
K-space View Reduction	
Reduced phase encodes	Resolution loss
Rectangular field of view	Not amenable to all anatomy
Parallel/compressed acquisition	SNR loss and potential artifacts
RF Pulses	
Reduced flip angle excite and/or refocus	SNR loss and contrast changes
Pulse amplitude/width modulation	SNR loss; sequence timing issues
Saturation/suppression pulse reduction	Contrast changes; artifacts
Time Efficiency	
Increase concatenations	Longer acquisition times
Reduce ETL; increase ESP and/or TR	Longer acquisition times
Reduce anatomic coverage	Need for multiple acquisitions
Increase slice thickness/spacing	Slice resolution loss
Pulse Sequence	
Gradient vs spin echo or bSSFP	Contrast and SNR considerations
RF Coil Selection or Patient Positioning	
Smaller volume transmit coils	Coverage, uniformity, availability

Note that increases in acquisition times add to motion problems and increase overall active scan times. Increasing RF pulse excitation may be more susceptible to both motion and relaxation effects.

Abbreviations: bSSFP, balanced steady-state free precession; ESP, echo spacing; ETL, echo train length; SNR, signal/noise ratio.

equal to 1°C increase in body core temperature are not expected to result in adverse health effects.[38] In persons at risk for thermoregulatory impairment (eg, infants, pregnant women, persons with cardiocirculatory impairment), the temperature increase should be less than or equal to 0.5°C. Maximum temperatures in localized regions should be managed as well for head (≤38°C), trunk (≤39°C), and limbs (≤40°C).

To prevent undue heat stress and tissue damage, the SAR output of the MR imaging is governed with the goal of limiting increases in local and whole-body temperature. Normal operating mode limits total body core or local temperature to less than or equal to 39°C and temperature changes to less than or equal to 0.5°C. First-level controlled operating mode limits total body core or local temperature to less than or equal to 40°C and temperature changes to less than or equal to 1°C.

In terms of how this translates to SAR limits, for volume transmit coils (ie, body, head, extremity), the whole-body SAR normal operating mode limit is 2 W/kg and for first-level controlled operating mode first-level controlled operating mode it is 4 W/kg.[10] Partial-body SAR ranges from those

whole-body limits up to 10 W/kg as the fraction of exposed tissue decreases, whereas SAR in the head specifically is limited to 3.2 W/kg for either operator mode. Local transmit coils have limits of 10 W/kg and 20 W/kg for normal and first-level controlled modes, respectively in the head and trunk and double these values for extremities. All limits are 6-minute averages, with the average in any 10-second window being less than twice the stated limit. In addition, with the higher SAR of local transmit coils, care needs to be taken with sensitive tissues in the field, such as the orbits of the eyes, to keep temperature increases less than 1°C. Exceeding the first-level controlled operating mode first-level controlled operating mode limits is only done within the confines of human-subject research studies.

Note that first-level controlled operating mode first-level controlled operating mode whole-body limits assumes patients have uncompromised thermoregulatory capability. Thermoregulatory capabilities can be compromised by the ambient room environment limiting heat exchange with the environment. The SAR limits assumed an ambient temperature of less than or equal to 25°C and less than or equal to 60% humidity. Whole-body SAR limits may be reduced by 0.25 W/kg per degree Celsius exceeding 25°C until SAR is returned to the normal operating mode limit.

MR examinations that expose more of the body over longer periods of time (eg, whole-body examinations, cervical-thoracic-lumbar spine examinations, combined abdomen-pelvic examinations, PET/MR imaging) have increased in frequency. To help balance the thermoregulatory stress in light of sustained power deposition, a simple active scan time metric for the total energy delivered to the patient has been developed for aiding in promoting best practices during these examinations by limiting, or giving patients time to recover between, long examination times.[10] The specific absorbed energy (SAE) is an estimate of the total energy delivered into the patient during the active scan time. The current recommended maximum SAE is 14.4 kJ/kg (or 240 W*min/kg). If followed, this SAE recommendation limits active scanning at the normal operating mode SAR limit of 2 W/kg to less than 120 minutes and for first-level controlled operating mode SAR limit of 4 W/kg to less than 60 minutes. If SAE limits are reached during an examination, different vendors may have different safety interlocks in place that can warn, or stop, the user. In any event, if the SAE is reached, it is recommended to check on the patient's status and potentially allow a period of time to cool down if needed.

Irreversible thermal tissue damage is a function of both temperature and exposure. Unless temperatures are very high (>57°C), damage takes seconds to minutes to develop. The primary mechanism to irreversible damage of tissue is denaturation of key proteins needed to maintain cellular hemostasis or membrane activity so that the rate of transition from the normal to damaged state (Ω) can be modeled as a function of temperature (T) via a first order Arrhenius rate[39]

$$\Omega = A \int_0^t e^{\frac{-E_a}{RT(\tau)}} d\tau \qquad \textbf{Equation 7}$$

where the estimated fraction of tissue in the damaged state (F_D) would be given by $F_D = 1 - e^{-\Omega}$, and R is the universal gas constant (8.3145 J/mol/K). The original work on high-temperature skin burns established a frequency factor $A = 3.1 \times 10^{98}$ s^{-1}, and $E_a = 6.28 \times 10^5$ J mol^{-1}is the activation energy for the process. Although these original parameters are still often used for predicting tissue damage at high temperatures, a tremendous amount of work has been performed

not only to refine the original values and identify temperature dependent breakpoints but to successfully adapt to different tissues and processes.[40,41] Pioneering work by Sapareto and Dewey[42] resulted in a simplified version of this model that is useful for hyperthermia dosimetry,[42,43] where many different isoeffects could be characterized simply by the characterizing the cumulative equivalent minutes spent at 43°C (CEM_{43}).

$$CEM_{43} = \sum_{t=0}^{n \cdot \Delta t} R^{(43-T_n)} \cdot \Delta t, \; with$$
$$R = \begin{cases} 0.25 & T_n < 43°C \\ 0.50 & T_n \geq 43°C \end{cases}$$

Equation 8

Here R is not the universal gas constant, but represents the rate of damage accumulation with time. Although values for R can vary, the most important result from a safety aspect is that at more than 43°C, damage begins to accumulate exponentially faster with dose and approximately doubles for each degree Celsius increase in temperature. Damage that takes 60 minutes to accumulate at 43°C, takes 15 minutes at 45°C or 4 hours at 42°C. Because of the exponential nature of this curve and the high uncertainty this introduces at low temperatures, application to assessing risk at higher temperatures, such as those associated with sustained focal heating, make thermal dosimetry a powerful compliment to modeling and measurement techniques, but not immediately useful with respect to controlling whole-body heating.[44,45]

It cannot be stressed enough that neither SAR limits nor SAE guidance have been developed with the prevention of RF burns in mind. These limits are designed to diminish discomfort from thermal stress or potential damage that can accumulate over long periods of exposure time with slow heating. Heating rate is proportional to SAR, and so the high SAR associated with focal heating can result in much faster increases in temperature. Unlike diffuse heating of the patient that leads to discomfort, focal heating may heat locations where the patient is less sensitive to the pain, or at very fast rates, such that patient monitoring based on verbal feedback or the bulb to stop the scan may be ineffective. Therefore, prevention of focal heating in the patient is an important separate consideration. The potential for focal heating in routine MR imaging has a strong dependence on proper patient screening, preparation, and positioning, as well as appropriate management of what materials or devices accompany the patient into the scanner.

Radiofrequency-Induced Focal Heating

Higher-caliber currents that may result in focal resistive heating in tissue can also be induced by the applied RF field and are a function of material conductivity, geometry, and location in the excitation coil. The primary concern along with these distributions of current are focal areas of high resistance that can lead to resistive heating of tissue. Materials with high conductivity, such as metals, tend to have current density highest at the surface. For smaller conducting materials (<2 cm) there is not a high probability of significant heating unless there are adjacent conductors within about 3 cm that may couple for enhanced heating.[46] Larger conductors, such as a hip or spine prosthetic, can generate a significant amount of current. If the object is large and smooth, these currents tend to distribute uniformly across the material, spreading the energy over a large volume. Medical implants, such as a drug infusion pump, result in heating distributed across their volume, which can be managed. However, at sharp corners or disconnects, or when in close proximity to another conductor, there is potential for high electric fields and resistive heating in the adjacent tissue.

Conducting loops

One specific geometry that presents risks in MR imaging is conductors forming loops in the RF field that are nearly perpendicular to the applied field. As discussed regarding Faraday's law, a time-varying magnetic field induces an electromotive force in these effective conducting loops generating a current proportional to the area of the loop and magnetic flux. Larger loops result in larger induced currents. This current, and hence the heating, will be distributed all along the loop if there are no areas of high resistance. However, areas of high resistance, such as breaks in the loop, will generate hotspots where this large current can be turned into heat, which can be substantial. In some cases, the electrical properties of the loop have a resonance frequency close to the Larmor frequency, in which a very large amount of current can be generated. Although it is unlikely for a random conducting loop to be near resonance in the RF field, the receive array coils are designed to be at resonance and are actively blanked during transmit. Because of the potential of surface coils to heat during imaging, vendors design and test coils in both connected and unconnected modes. In general, temperatures should not exceed 41°C.[10,47]

Of course, metal is not the only conductor in the magnet capable of high-caliber current loops. Human skin and/or damp clothing can also be highly conductive. The clasping of hands can form a large-diameter conducting loop from the arms, chest, and shoulders. The point of contact (ie, fingers or hands) is a potential region of high resistance where rapid, high heating can occur.[48] Similarly, crossing of legs (ankle to ankle or calf to calf), hands to outer thighs, or inner thigh to thigh contact have been associated with RF-induced thermal injury. Next to direct contact with external conductors, skin-to-skin contact is one of the most identified root causes for reported burns in MR scanners.[27]

Antenna effect

Long, cylindrical conductors, such as needles, wires, or leads, may be implanted, or partially implanted, in patients, and are additional sources of potential heating. For these objects, the induced tangential electric field drives the current density along the length of the conductor. As with loops, in general, the longer the length, the higher the potential current density and potential to deposit energy at a location of high resistance, such as the lead tip. Also as with a current loop, there is a resonance phenomenon in which the transfer of power from the RF field to the conductor is dramatically enhanced. In particular, when the object length is close to the half-wavelength of the RF field in tissue, the potential for very rapid and high heating exists (antenna effect).[49,50] As discussed earlier, the wavelength in tissue is reduced by the relative permittivity. However, there is an additional small loss for conductance that should be accounted for as well.[50,51] Therefore, the effects are highly tissue dependent. Using dielectric properties of muscle, which is relevant to implant locations, the half-wavelengths are approximately 20 cm (1.5 T) and 12 cm (3.0 T). The degree of heating can easily reach higher than 10°C in seconds, resulting in potential localized tissue damage early in an acquisition. In addition to this critical length effect and associated tissue dependence, for leads, the local temperature increase is a complex function of configuration, amount of material within tissue versus air, amount of insulation, as well as location in the RF coil. Implants closer to the edge of the coil tend to experience higher electric fields.

$B_1^+{}_{rms}$ and focal heating

Note that SAR operates as a dosimetric unit for diffuse heating over a large volume. However, because of the complexities that go into SAR prediction for these purposes, it does not track well with the extent of focal heating from a conductor in the RF field. For focal heating, estimated maximum $B_1^+{}_{rms}$, which might better relate to the maximum induced E_1 field and hence temperature, is a better output control variable. This output should be displayed on all MR scanners for helping to manage metal devices or implants that may be in the field.[10]

With this in mind, whether SAR or $B_1{}^+{}_{rms}$ is used for RF output control in the presence of conducting passive or active implants or external devices, primary guidance comes from standardized testing of these objects, which may include both theoretic and empirical results.[17,25,52,53] Just as with static field force effects being dependent on the magnet design, it is important to understand the limitations of the testing conditions for RF heating. Higher field (>3 T) scanners now routinely use 2-channel or higher transmit body coils in order to better tailor the RF transmission field to the size and shape of the anatomy of interest. The changes in amplitude and phase associated with these techniques have not been applied to the device being tested to assess the MR conditions in the MR scanner. In addition, lower field vertical magnets also orient the RF field in a different direction than the assumed direction of the implant and can have a very different (favorable or unfavorable) effect on the heating.[54] For these reasons, considerations of the conditions under which an assessment of safe conditions for MR scanning has been made should be considered when a conducting device is being considered for scanning.

Summary of Radiofrequency Safety in Magnetic Resonance Imaging

The primary risk associated with the time-varying RF magnetic field in MR imaging is tissue heating from absorption of currents induced during excitation. For the RF energy delivered to patients in routine MR imaging, these currents are distributed widely over the patient volume, resulting in diffuse heating that may lead to uncomfortable thermal stress to the patient. The increase in body core temperature is primarily controlled by regulating the dosimetry output of SAR, which approximates the power delivered to the patient, and monitoring the patient during the exposure. Long exposures may require breaks and time to cool off, and patients should be visually and audibly monitored. In addition, the temperature, humidity, and air flow in the MR scanner can influence the ability of patients to dissipate heat. Some patients are at risk because of conditions that may compromise their thermoregulatory capability, or ability to feel or report issues. A summary of these considerations is given in **Table 3**A. These patients may require additional medical supervision and

appropriate monitoring to manage risks from these stresses, such as ECG monitoring for cardiovascular stress.

The induced current density can also become concentrated in regions of higher resistance, resulting in higher temperature focal heating that can lead to irreversible tissue damage (ie, burns) when certain configurations of conductors are present. This focal heating is the leading cause of reported injuries in the MR environment. Neither the SAR output control nor exposure considerations are designed to prevent these thermal events. In addition, damage may happen so quickly that the patient is not able to report a problem until it is too late. Avoiding these thermal events is primarily a matter of proper patient screening for conducting objects and implants; mindful patient and conducting device positioning to avoid and insulate contact between any conducting surfaces, including the MR equipment and patient themselves; as well as avoiding exposures of these conductors to high B_1 hotspots near the transmitting coil (ie, bore wall) (**Fig. 3**). A summary of the consideration for focal heating is also provided in **Table 3**B.

Conducting passive implanted medical devices or AIMDs are of particular concern for heating. In addition, the RF field may induce unintended stimulation as well as temporary or permanent device malfunction for certain AIMDs.[25] Methodologies for empirical and model-based testing to help characterize conditions for safe scanning of these devices have evolved substantially over time and many specific devices, or device groups, have some form of guidelines with conditions under the control of the user by which both patient and device can be appropriately managed for RF heating in the MR environment.

As MR technology evolves, such as the move toward higher fields and multitransmit technologies, as well as a greater variety of devices being implanted in patients in order to manage conditions associated with, among other things, chronic disease and extended life span, understanding and keeping current with the physics and technology associated with RF heating by practitioners of MR imaging is paramount to maintaining and steadily improving the overall safety profile that continues to provide increasing patient access to this critical technology for managing their care.

Time-Varying Gradient Magnetic Field

During pulse sequencing, additional coils within the bore are used to create time-varying gradient magnetic fields for image encoding purposes.

Table 3
Summary of radiofrequency heating risk factors for patients

RF Heating Risk	Risk Factors
Whole-body or Partial-body Heating[a]	
Environment	• Bore temperature (ideally $\leq$22°C; not to exceed 25°C) • Humidity should be maintained $\leq$60% • Unobstructed air flow in bore (fan)
Patient	• Compromised thermoregulatory capability • Fever, cardiac decompensation, inability to perspire, hypertension, diabetes, obesity, elderly, certain patients with cancer • Pregnant patients, neonates, and low-birth-weight infants • Medications (eg, diuretics, β-blockers, calcium blockers, amphetamines, sedatives,) • Avoid thermal insulation (eg, heavy clothing, blankets) • Unconscious, sedated, or loss of feeling in any body part • Appropriate patient monitoring plan
RF exposure	• High SAR for sustained period • Single acquisition >15 min • Active scan time examination >60 min
Focal Heating	
Patient preparation	• Electrical insulation between patient and any conductors • Patient isolated from bore, RF coils and cables, and skin-to-skin contact via vendor-recommended padding • RF coils, cables, and leads isolated from bore wall and each other • All coils/leads properly engaged (ie, plugged in) • Use only properly maintained, operated, and undamaged MR conditional equipment • Uncommunicative and/or anesthetized patients • Appropriate patient monitoring plan
Conductors	• Avoid unnecessary conductors and/or metallic objects • Damp clothing, diapers, hair or skin • Jewelry, tattoos, makeup, hair products, clothing • Medicinal transdermal patches • Active, passive, or on-body implanted medical devices • Read and follow MR conditions on all devices or implants • Metallic objects as far from bore wall as possible • Two or more conductors in close proximity ($\leq$3 cm)
Current loops	• Avoid circular, U-shaped, S-shaped conductor configurations • Skin-to-skin contact • Coil cables and conducting leads • Tattoos • Jewelry
Antenna effect	• Elongated implants, including fully or partially implanted leads, interventional needles, and guidewires • Greatest risks near resonant length or longer
RF exposure	• High SAR for short or sustained periods • Use lowest possible SAR

[a] Consider restricting to normal operator mode and/or use appropriate medical supervision and patient monitoring if risk factors cannot be mitigated.

The coils seek to modulate the value of the axial (B_z) by an amount small with respect to the magnetic field (mT) linearly around isocenter of each logical axis (x, y, z). These gradient magnetic fields (G_x, G_y, G_z) range from their lowest value at the isocenter to their largest positive or negative values near the edge of the usable field of view in each direction. Gradients in each direction can be run simultaneously, providing for a rapid change in the local magnetic field (dB/dt) at points away from the isocenter. The rapid switching of these gradients during acquisitions and associated dB/

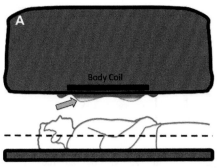
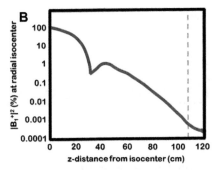

Fig. 3. Spatial distribution of RF power in MR imaging. The internal whole-body volume transmit-receive coil is the primary source for RF excitation in modern MR imaging. The coil is usually a multirung birdcage quadrature coil. Near the edge of the bore, the RF field intensity can be large (*A*), with the highest intensity occurring near the edge of the coil in the z-direction away from isocenter. Because the rungs are configured in a circle around the bore, these hotspots occur periodically around the bore as well, which can be a safety concern for patient anatomy (especially upper extremities or shoulders), devices, and/or medical implants abutted up against the edge of the bore and not protected by proper padding as recommended by the vendor. Vendor-supplied documents on the spatial distribution of the RF field (*B*) show the transmitted RF power along the magnet isocenter and do not include these hot spots. However, such plots are still useful for estimating the exposure to a particular region of anatomy, device, or implant in the field. RF power decreases to less than 1% at the edge of the coil (approximately z = 30 cm for this system) and is many decades attenuated by the edge of the bore (*gray dashed line*). Therefore, although the highest RF power experienced by most tissue lies near isocenter, hotspots at the radial edge of the bore wall must be considered for patients and devices in these areas.

dt away from the isocenter is responsible for the primary safety concerns from this field[55] because this generates the loud acoustic noise associated with MR imaging; can induce potentially uncomfortable nerve stimulation in the patient; or, in the case of AIMDs in particular, may result in unintended stimulation to the patient, device vibration and heating, as well as temporary disruption or permanent damage to the device.[25]

Powerful gradients are a hallmark of modern MR scanners because they facilitate rapid, high-resolution volume imaging and shorter echo times and echo spacing, among other performance enhancements. Large currents (kiloamps) are switched on the gradient coils in the bore to generate the linear magnetic field in each direction. Generating this amount of current results in significant equipment heating, which requires active cooling of the system. Imaging when the cooling system is not fully functional can result in overheating and permanent damage. Gradient performance is generally characterized by the maximum amplitude per axis (40–80 mT), fastest increase time (100–400 microseconds), and maximum slew rate (130–200 T/m/s). These values are usually part of standard gradient performance specifications provided by the vendor in describing the system and can be useful for characterizing the system, although the stated specifications may exceed what the system can actually apply during routine imaging because of safety or system gradient heating limitations.

As the gradients switch on and off during an acquisition, the associated dB/dt is largest away from the isocenter (**Fig. 4**), and it is near these locations that safety concerns with respect to interaction with patients and devices are greatest. In particular, the largest potential value when all gradients are simultaneously at maximum slew happens at a location away from the z-isocenter, near the edge of the bore. The spatial distribution of these values (T/s) for making safety decisions can be found in the vendor system manual.

Peripheral Nerve Stimulation

As previously discussed, time-varying magnetic fields result in an electromotive force and resulting electric field in conducting materials via Faradays' law of induction. Time-varying gradients differ from RF in that dB/dt has a higher amplitude but a much lower frequency (kilohertz). However, even the systems with the weakest gradients on the market are capable of exceeding the stimulation threshold for the tissue. The system operating mode safety limits have been developed to limit this peripheral nerve stimulation (PNS), which may result in patient discomfort. Beyond comfort, it is important to limit PNS because examination efficacy can be compromised by movement associated with this patient discomfort or agitation. In addition, PNS thresholds in the current region of operation have also been shown to be below cardiac stimulation thresholds, which could result in

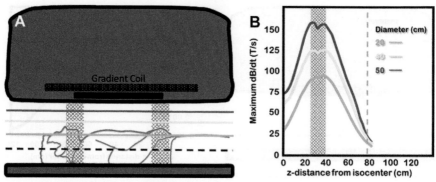

Fig. 4. The distribution of maximum gradient magnetic field dB/dt in MR imaging. A patient lying in an MR scanner (*A*) experiences increasing dB/dt as a function of radial distance from isocenter. Here, radii for diameters around isocenter are shown for 20 cm (*green*), 40 cm (*yellow*), and 50 cm (*green*). When combined with the increasing dB/dt in the z-direction moving away from isocenter, the maximum dB/dt the patient can experience happens in the cross-hatched regions near the edge of the gradient coil. These large dB/dt may be the source of painful stimulation or could damage/disrupt AIMDs in the patient. A plot of these regions for a 60-cm diameter bore magnet with powerful gradients (80 mT/m amplitude and 200 T/m/s slew rate) is also shown (*B*).

additional patient safety events, such as induced arrhythmia.

PNS is characterized by tingling sensations of slight muscle spasms in the ribs, side, abdomen, hip, buttock, or thoracic regions, or along the upper arms or the back muscles in the shoulder region. There is a large variance in stimulation thresholds in patients depending on physiologic conditions. In addition, the specific coil design and gradient pulse shapes are factors as well. As opposed to using derived values, stimulation limits for a specific system can be determined by averaging the individual stimulation thresholds of test subjects. First-level controlled operating mode is such that 50% of all patients experience at least mild stimulations after reaching the stimulation threshold. Normal operating mode limits the scanner to 80% of this threshold.

Mathematically maximum magnetic field switching threshold for PNS can be modeled as a hyperbolic function[55]:

$$\left.\frac{dB}{dt}\right|_{max} = b\left(1 + \frac{c}{d}\right)$$

Equation 9

Where b is the mean threshold for stimulation (rheobase) given an infinite pulse duration, and c is the duration at which the stimulation threshold is twice the rheobase. Chronaxie is the smallest time duration required for stimulation for an amplitude twice the rheobase, and d is the pulse duration ($d = 2 \cdot G_{max}/G_{slew}$ for trapezoidal gradients). In general, greater stimulus strengths result in shorter stimulation times. This hyperbolic form for stimulation threshold best fits data from both early numerical simulation work and experimental data.[56-58]

From a fit of the data, threshold output values for PNS on whole-body gradient systems are a rheobase of 20 T/s for first-level operator mode and chronaxie of 0.36 milliseconds. The rheobase is reduced by 80% for normal operator mode. If the vendor has gradients capable of a rheobase higher than 20 T/s, then further testing is needed to establish stimulation thresholds.[15] Hardware is ultimately limited by the 1% cardiac threshold ($c = 3$ milliseconds and $b = 20$ T/s) derived from simulation with a safety factor of 3 reducing the cardiac rheobase such that risk of cardiac stimulations at higher ramp times is reduced.[10]

Time-Varying Magnetic Fields and Medical Devices

In the presence of a conducting medical device or implant, rapid switching (dB/dt) of powerful gradients is a consideration.[25] Heating of conducting devices was covered previously for RF pulses. With gradient pulses, the instantaneous power deposited by the eddy currents from the switched gradient field can lead to device heating. Power is estimated similar to Equation 6, but with dB/dt replacing $f \cdot B_1$, making heating proportional to the product of the conductivity, volume, and |dB/dt|.[2] Most notably, these effects likely only come into play near the regions of maximum dB/dt for large-volume implants. Vibration can arise from gradient switching because of an eddy current–induced magnetic moment attempting to align with the static field. The induced torque (L) is similar to Equation 3 and is the product of the conductivity, volume, static field, and dB/dt. In addition, for AIMDs, there is the potential for unintended patient stimulation from induced voltages on leads, and device malfunction, such as device malfunction caused by electrical interference. As with SAR, the calculations of dB/dt provided by the vendor are provided for estimating likelihood of PNS, not for establishing and adhering to thresholds for interactions with implanted or external devices.[25]

Gradient-Induced Acoustic Noise

A current-carrying coil in a strong static magnetic field experiences a force (Lorentz) orthogonal to both the current and the magnetic field. This movement of the coil during gradient slewing is the primary source of acoustic noise in MR scanners.[59,60] Because the noise may be uncomfortable, cause anxiety, or result in temporary hearing loss for patients, vendors work hard to design gradients in which the acoustic noise generated from these mechanical forces is minimized. The physical aspects of acoustic noise are characterized by the frequency spectrum, intensity, and duration of exposure.

Measurements are made versus a reference acoustic pressure value (p_0), such as the threshold for human hearing (20 µPa at 1 kHz). The peak allowable sound pressure level (SPL) when referenced against the lowest sound pressure is given by:

$$SPL(dB) = 20 \, log_{10}\left(\frac{p}{p_0}\right) \qquad \textbf{Equation 10}$$

Peak average SPL exposure for adults is 140 dB (eg, jet engine) and 120 dB for children. Because human hearing is sensitive in a particular part of the audio frequency spectrum, time-limited exposure limits tend to be weighted to emphasize measurement of noise in this part of the audio spectrum (approximately 1–8 kHz) as the human ear might, and hence the SPL is designated as the A-weighted average (dB-A). The IEC limit for patients in MR imaging is less than or equal to 99 dB-A, extrapolated from World Health Organization (WHO) occupational exposures, under the constraining assumption of a single exposure in a day for 1 hour.[10] This value may be increased or decreased by 3 dB-A for halving or doubling of the exposure time, respectively.

In general, noise levels in the bore average around 115 dB-A and can reach peaks of 135 dB-A, with fast sequences, such as echoplanar imaging (EPI), generally being the loudest. At the console, the levels are usually less than 60 dB-A. Therefore, hearing protection should be used to decrease noise to at least 99 dB-A for patients and 85 dB-A for personnel in the examination room[61] via hearing protection (ie, plugs,

muffs, or both) with noise reduction ratings greater than 29 dB. Note that, because the noise reduction ratio stated depends on proper placement, it is extremely important to make certain that personnel are properly trained in placing and checking placement of these devices in the various clinical scenarios, such as children, neonates, or anesthetized patients. In addition, an array of quiet or silent sequences has become available from vendors. These sequences often come with a tradeoff between desired timing, contrast, and/or signal/noise ratio. In the end, the established guidelines reflect a continuous exposure, whereas it is unlikely that maximal acoustic noise exposure would be present during the entire time spent on the table.

Safety Concerns of Time-Varying Gradient Magnetic Field Summary

The primary safety concerns arising from the time-varying gradient magnetic field arise from dB/dt, which is responsible for generating the loud acoustic noise associated with MR imaging that mandates hearing protection be used when in the suite during imaging procedures.

Another safety concern is the potentially for uncomfortable PNS when operating in the first-level operating mode. The likelihood of experiencing stimulation is greatly reduced in normal operating mode where gradient performance is derated to 80% of maximum.

In addition, the impact of the gradient magnetic field on implants can result in heating, vibration, unintended patient stimulation, or active device malfunctions. These conditions may also require the system be run in normal operating mode, restriction of positioning of the device within the bore during imaging, or in the future using vendor ability to use the IEC fixed-parameter option for gradients,[10,25] similar to how some vendors have allowed use of a fixed SAR or $B_1{}^+_{rms}$ below the normal operating mode limit.

High-performance sequences tend to use large dB/dt gradient pulses, such as EPI, which are used for diffusion or functional MR imaging examinations, as well as balanced steady-state free precession acquisitions, which require rapid, short-TR and short-echo-time (TE) acquisitions for applications such as real-time or CINE cardiac acquisitions. Note that running the MR system in normal operating mode for dB/dt may affect high-performance acquisitions. The speed of acquisitions (including breath-hold times), slice and/or in-plane resolution, and contrast caused by potential increases in echo-spacing or minimum TE (ie, echo-trains, Dixon imaging, in-phase/out-of-phase imaging) may all be modified and require some attention to ensure the quality and completion of the examination. As gradient performance continues to be pushed, using novel gradient coil or pulse design, and better modeling of patient stimulation or device interactions, it may aid in maintaining both patient safety and access to high-performance acquisitions for a large population of patients.

DISCUSSION

MR imaging has been one of the fastest-proliferating advanced imaging modalities in medical imaging. Despite the rapid growth in both use and technology, MR imaging remains one of the safest advanced imaging services available. In addition, when operated within the established regulated output parameters by knowledgeable teams of personnel who remain diligent and up to date in their MR safety training, MR imaging also remains a nonsignificant medical device according to the FDA.

As shown in this article, the primary safety concerns in the MR environment arise from the physical consequences of the presence of the static magnetic field, which is always on for high-field systems, and the time-varying RF and gradient magnetic fields, which are active during image acquisition. Advances in MR technology, such as higher-field-strength systems with more powerful gradients, remain within the regulated output parameters but may introduce new issues regarding patient safety that require constant vigilance by the MR teams managing the patients. These teams must understand the impact of changes in the technology, including under what circumstances and to what degree patient management may need to change in order to maintain patient safety for a given system.

Knowledge of the basic potential interactions between the patients, devices, and the MR scanner facilitates more informed and timely patient management decisions that help to maintain patient access to MR imaging. This process may increasingly include routing of patients to specific systems with an safety profile amenable to their particular needs and medical conditions, or to manage MR safety conditions on an implanted device. To accomplish this, it is imperative to be able to assess and understand the safety parameters of the MR system and the specific conditions needed to successfully complete an examination while managing the risks.

In the presence of increasing numbers of implantable medical devices, wearable technology, and other devices being tested to establish highly specific conditions for managing the risks associated with scanning in MR imaging, knowledge of field strength and operating mode restrictions is no longer enough. Users must understand the output and output distribution of which their system is capable, how these relate to the management of their patients, and the tools or procedures for controlling exposures on their systems. Artifacts, or the changes needed to manage the patients, may affect diagnostic quality of the examination, especially those examinations relying on high-performance acquisitions. With this in mind, reassessing the appropriateness of the MR examination, and how to modify the examination to achieve the needed goals safely, are skills that will be important for the team to have to maintain appropriate patient access to this advanced imaging service. Understanding the potential issues and tradeoffs in MR imaging can aid teams in providing higher-reliability examination safety and quality through more informed patient selection, protocoling, screening, scanning, and interpretation.

Clinics care points

- An understanding of the physical underpinnings of MRI safety is necessary for informed risk-benefit decision making as well as risk management.

- Applying the physical principles of MRI safety to the management of patients in the MR environment as well as acquisition protocols can aid in reducing patient discomfort, enhancing both patient compliance and image quality as well as safety.

DISCLOSURE

The authors have nothing to disclose.

REFERENCES

1. Expert Panel on MRS, Kanal E, Barkovich AJ, et al. ACR guidance document on MR safe practices: 2013. J Magn Reson Imaging 2013;37(3):501–30.
2. ACR Committee on MR Safety:, Greenberg TD, Hoff MN, Gilk TB, et al. ACR guidance document on MR safe practices: Updates and critical information 2019. J Magn Reson Imaging 2020;51(2):331–8.
3. Panych LP, Madore B. The physics of MRI safety. J Magn Reson Imaging 2018;47(1):28–43.
4. Nyenhuis JA, Park SM, Kamondetdacha R, et al. MRI and implanted medical devices: Basic interactions with an emphasis on heating. IEEE Trans Device Mater Reliab 2005;5(3):467–80.
5. Hoff MN, McKinney At, Shellock FG, et al. Safety Considerations of 7-T MRI in Clinical Practice. Radiology 2019;292(3):509–18.

6. Tsai LL, Grant AK, Mortele KJ, et al. A Practical Guide to MR Imaging Safety: What Radiologists Need to Know. Radiographics 2015;35(6): 1722–37.

7. McRobbie DW. Occupational exposure in MRI. Br J Radiol 2012;85(1012):293–312.

8. Schenck JF. The role of magnetic susceptibility in magnetic resonance imaging: MRI magnetic compatibility of the first and second kinds. Med Phys 1996;23(6):815–50.

9. Schenck JF. Safety of strong, static magnetic fields. J Magn Reson Imaging 2000;12(1):2–19.

10. IEC. IEC 60601-60602-33: particular requirements for the basic safety and essential performance of magnetic resonance diagnostic equipment. Geneva (Switzerland): IEC; 2015.

11. ASTM F2052 standard test method for measurement of magnetically induced displacement force on medical devices in the magnetic resonance environment. West Conshohocken (PA): ASTM International; 2015.

12. Shellock FG, Kanal E, Gilk TB. Regarding the value reported for the term "spatial gradient magnetic field" and how this information is applied to labeling of medical implants and devices. AJR Am J Roentgenol 2011;196(1):142–5.

13. Woods TO, Delfino JG, Shein MJ. Response to Standardized MR Terminology and Reporting of Implants and Devices as Recommended by the American College of Radiology Subcommittee on MR Safety. Radiology 2016;279(3):906–9.

14. Kanal E, Froelich J, Barkovich AJ, et al. Standardized MR terminology and reporting of implants and devices as recommended by the American College of Radiology Subcommittee on MR Safety. Radiology 2015;274(3):866–70.

15. Administration USFD. Submission of premarket notifications for magnetic resonance diagnostic devices: guidance for industry and Food and Drug Administration staff. Silver Spring (MD): U.S. Food & Drug Administration; 2016.

16. ASTM F2213 standard test method for measurement of magnetically induced torque on medical devices in the magnetic resonance environment. West Conshohocken (PA): ASTM International; 2017.

17. Administration USFD. Testing and labeling medical devices for safety in the magnetic resonance (MR) environment: draft guidance for industry and Food and Drug Administration Staff. Silver Spring (MD): U.S. Food & Drug Administration; 2019.

18. Condon B, Hadley DM. Potential MR hazard to patients with metallic heart valves: the Lenz effect. J Magn Reson Imaging 2000;12(1):171–6.

19. Edwards MB, McLean J, Solomonidis S, et al. In vitro assessment of the Lenz effect on heart valve prostheses at 1.5 T. J Magn Reson Imaging 2015; 41(1):74–82.

20. Schenck JF. Physical interactions of static magnetic fields with living tissues. Prog Biophys Mol Biol 2005;87(2–3):185–204.

21. WHO. Environmental health Criteria 232: static fields. Geneva (Switzerland): World Health Organization; 2006.

22. International Commission on Non-Ionizing Radiation, Protection. Guidelines for limiting exposure to electric fields induced by movement of the human body in a static magnetic field and by time-varying magnetic fields below 1 Hz. Health Phys 2014; 106(3):418–25.

23. Kinouchi Y, Yamaguchi H, Tenforde TS. Theoretical analysis of magnetic field interactions with aortic blood flow. Bioelectromagnetics 1996; 17(1):21–32.

24. Administration USFD. Criteria for significant risk investigations of magnetic resonance diagnostic devices - guidance for industry and Food and Drug Administration Staff. Silver Spring (MD): U.S. Food & Drug Administration; 2014.

25. (ISO) IOfS. ISO/TS 10974: assessment of the safety of magnetic resonance imaging for patients with an active implantable medical device. Geneva (Switzerland): International Organization for Standardization (ISO); 2018.

26. Indik JH, Gimbel JR, Abe H, et al. 2017 HRS expert consensus statement on magnetic resonance imaging and radiation exposure in patients with cardiovascular implantable electronic devices. Heart Rhythm 2017;14(7):e97–153.

27. Delfino JG, Krainak DM, Flesher SA, et al. MRI-related FDA adverse event reports: A 10-yr review. Med Phys 2019;46(12):5562–71.

28. Shellock FG. Radiofrequency energy-induced heating during MR procedures: a review. J Magn Reson Imaging 2000;12(1):30–6.

29. Gabriel S, Lau RW, Gabriel C. The dielectric properties of biological tissues: II. Measurements in the frequency range 10 Hz to 20 GHz. Phys Med Biol 1996; 41(11):2251–69.

30. Murbach M, Neufeld E, Cabot E, et al. Virtual population-based assessment of the impact of 3 Tesla radiofrequency shimming and thermoregulation on safety and B1 + uniformity. Magn Reson Med 2016;76(3):986–97.

31. Murbach M, Neufeld E, Capstick M, et al. Thermal tissue damage model analyzed for different whole-body SAR and scan durations for standard MR body coils. Magn Reson Med 2014;71(1):421–31.

32. Nordbeck P, Fidler F, Weiss I, et al. Spatial distribution of RF-induced E-fields and implant heating in MRI. Magn Reson Med 2008;60(2):312–9.

33. Wang Z, Lin JC, Vaughan JT, et al. Consideration of physiological response in numerical models of temperature during MRI of the human head. J Magn Reson Imaging 2008;28(5):1303–8.

34. Iacono MI, Neufeld E, Akinnagbe E, et al. MIDA: A Multimodal Imaging-Based Detailed Anatomical Model of the Human Head and Neck. PLoS One 2015;10(4):e0124126.

35. National Electrical Manufacturers Association. NEMA MS 8 - characterization of the specific absorption rate (SAR) for magnetic resonance imaging systems. Association of Electrical Equipment and Medical Imaging Manufacturers. Rosslyn (VA): National Electrical Manufacturers Association; 2016.

36. Shellock F. Magnetic resonance procedures: health effects & safety. Boca Raton (FL): CRC Press; 2000.

37. National Electrical Manufacturers Association. NEMA MS 10 - determination of local specific absorption rate (SAR) in diagnostic magnetic resonance imaging. Association of Electrical Equipment and Medical Imaging Manufacturers. Rosslyn (VA): National Electrical Manufacturers Association; 2010.

38. International Commission on Non-Ionizing Radiation, Protection. Amendment to the ICNIRP "Statement on medical magnetic resonance (MR) procedures: protection of patients. Health Phys 2009;97(3):259–61.

39. Henriques FC, Moritz AR. Studies of Thermal Injury: I. The Conduction of Heat to and through Skin and the Temperatures Attained Therein. A Theoretical and an Experimental Investigation. Am J Pathol 1947;23(4):530–49.

40. Pearce JA. Comparative analysis of mathematical models of cell death and thermal damage processes. Int J Hyperthermia 2013;29(4):262–80.

41. Despa F, Orgill DP, Neuwalder J, et al. The relative thermal stability of tissue macromolecules and cellular structure in burn injury. Burns 2005;31(5):568–77.

42. Sapareto SA, Dewey WC. Thermal dose determination in cancer therapy. Int J Radiat Oncol Biol Phys 1984;10(6):787–800.

43. Dewey WC. Arrhenius relationships from the molecule and cell to the clinic. Int J Hyperthermia 1994; 10(4):457–83.

44. Sienkiewicz Z, van Rongen E, Croft R, et al. A Closer Look at the Thresholds of Thermal Damage: Workshop Report by an ICNIRP Task Group. Health Phys 2016;111(3):300–6.

45. van Rhoon GC, Samaras T, Yarmolenko PS, et al. CEM43°C thermal dose thresholds: a potential guide for magnetic resonance radiofrequency exposure levels? Eur Radiol 2013;23(8):2215–27.

46. Song T, Xu Z, Iacono MI, et al. Retrospective analysis of RF heating measurements of passive medical implants. Magn Reson Med 2018;80(6):2726–30.

47. IEC.. IEC 60601-1-11: medical electrical equipment — Part 1-11: general requirements for basic safety and essential performance — Collateral standard: requirements for medical electrical equipment and medical electrical systems used in the home healthcare environment. Geneva (Switzerland): IEC; 2015.

48. Knopp MV, Essig M, Debus J, et al. Unusual burns of the lower extremities caused by a closed conducting loop in a patient at MR imaging. Radiology 1996;200(2):572–5.

49. Kainz W. MR heating tests of MR critical implants. J Magn Reson Imaging 2007;26(3):450–1.

50. Bennett MC, Wiant DB, Gersh JA, et al. Mechanisms and prevention of thermal injury from gamma radiosurgery headframes during 3T MR imaging. J Appl Clin Med Phys 2012;13(4):3613.

51. IEC. IEC/IEEE 62704-1: determining the peak spatial-average specific absorption rate (SAR) in the human body from wireless communications devices, 30 MHz to 6 GHz – Part 1: general requirements for using the finite-difference time-domain (FDTD) method for SAR calculations. Geneva (Switzerland): IEC; 2017.

52. International A. ASTM F2182-19e1, Standard Test Method for Measurement of Radio Frequency Induced Heating On or Near Passive Implants During Magnetic Resonance Imaging. West Conshohocken (PA): ASTM International; 2019.

53. Administration USFD. Establishing safety and compatibility of passive implants in the magnetic resonance (MR) environment: guidance for Industry and Food and Drug Administration staff. Silver Spring (MD): U.S. Food & Drug Administration; 2014.

54. Golestanirad L, Kazemivalipour E, Lampman D, et al. RF heating of deep brain stimulation implants in open-bore vertical MRI systems: A simulation study with realistic device configurations. Magn Reson Med 2020;83(6):2284–92.

55. Schaefer DJ, Bourland JD, Nyenhuis JA. Review of patient safety in time-varying gradient fields. J Magn Reson Imaging 2000;12(1):20–9.

56. Reilly JP. Principles of nerve and heart excitation by time-varying magnetic fields. NY Acad of Sci 1992; 649:96–117.

57. Schaefer DJ. Safety aspects of radio frequency power deposition. Magn Reson Imaging Clin N Am 1998;6(4):775–89.

58. Bourland JD, Nyenhuis JA, Schaefer DJ. Physiologic effects of intense MR imaging gradient fields. Neuroimaging Clin N Am 1999;9(2):363–77.

59. McJury M, Shellock FG. Auditory noise associated with MR procedures: a review. J Magn Reson Imaging 2000;12(1):37–45.

60. Moelker A, Maas RA, Lethimonnier F, et al. Interventional MR imaging at 1.5 T: quantification of sound exposure. Radiology 2002;224(3):889–95.

61. Manufacturers AoEEaMI. NEMA MS 4 - acoustic noise measurement procedure for diagnostic magnetic resonance imaging devices: association of electrical equipment and medical imaging manufacturers. Rosslyn (VA): National Electrical Manufacturers Association; 2010.

Standardized Approaches to MR Safety Assessment of Patients with Implanted Devices

Emanuel Kanal, MD, FISMRM, MRMD, MRSE

KEYWORDS

- MR imaging • Safety • MR safety • Standardization • Magnetic fields • RF fields
- Gradient magnetic fields

KEY POINTS

- MR imaging is unique in that instead of using only 1 energy source, 3 distinct fields/energy sources are used to generate every MR imaging image/study.
- Each field/energy source is associated with its own unique safety risk(s) for humans, especially for those in whom there are implanted devices or foreign bodies.
- Each field/energy source, and therefore attendant risk potentials, is located within the MR scanner and patient in a spatial distribution pattern that is (a) not homogeneous and (b) unique to each field/energy source.
- The location of greatest risk associated with a given MR imaging field or energy source can be physically quite remote from the anatomy being imaged.
- A standardized approach to assessing and even beginning to quantify risk of a device/foreign body patient undergoing an MR imaging examination is achievable and is outlined in this article.

INTRODUCTION

For more than a century, diagnostic radiology has been based primarily for taking a radiograph energy source and directing it so that at least part of the radiographs produced by this source would irradiate an anatomic region to be evaluated. Some of the radiograph photons shined at the anatomic region of interest would be absorbed, reflected, and/or deflected predominantly by the electrons within the tissues so irradiated. Others managed to successfully pass through the irradiated tissues unscathed. The greater the number of radiograph photographs that successfully struck the receiver on the other side of the patient being studied, the blacker that region of the image would appear, and vice versa. In this fashion, we would probe predominantly relative electron density on all radiograph-based studies. Anatomy with greater relative electron density, such as electron-rich bone or iodine-containing contrast agents, would appear whiter, whereas electron-poor regions, such as lung and air, would appear darker.

There are several known risks associated with exposure to ionizing radiation, with the dominant one being the potential to induce mutations/carcinogenesis. One way that diagnostic radiology manages this risk is to routinely only expose the anatomy to be examined to such ionizing radiation. For example, in the process of acquiring a chest radiograph, the transmitted energy is collimated in such a way as to only irradiate or expose the chest to this ionizing radiograph beam. Although the target volume to be examined is

---

Division of Emergency Radiology and Teleradiology, Magnetic Resonance Services, Department of Radiology, University of Pittsburgh Medical Center, East Wing, Suite 200, 200 Lothrop Street, Pittsburgh, PA 15213, USA
E-mail address: ekanal@pitt.edu

Magn Reson Imaging Clin N Am 28 (2020) 537–548
https://doi.org/10.1016/j.mric.2020.07.003
1064-9689/20/© 2020 Elsevier Inc. All rights reserved.

indeed exposed to this energy, collimation ensures minimal to no significant exposure to, for example, the radiograph-sensitive gonads while acquiring that chest radiograph.

Also inherent to such radiograph studies is the fact that the region that IS exposed to ionizing radiation is quite homogeneously exposed, such that the sides and middle of the irradiated volume are exposed to very similar levels of ionizing radiation, in both in energy levels (kV) and quantity/duration (mA·s). Furthermore, it is obvious to all that there is no "exposure" of the patient to this ionizing radiation unless we are actively "taking the picture." Before and after the actual "exposure," there are no ionizing radiation safety considerations associated with the (inactive) radiograph equipment.

This comfortable and familiar model has been integrally associated with diagnostic radiologists since our specialty began over a century ago. One energy source, one associated set of risks from that energy exposure, homogeneous irradiation of (and only of) the anatomy to be evaluated, any associated potential risks are restricted to (and only to) the tissue being examined, and of course the patient's tissues are only exposed to this diagnostic energy while the system is activated for diagnostic imaging purposes. Between patients, there is no such energy produced, because the energy source is inactive, and therefore, no associated risks about which to be concerned.

It is precisely this clean, neat, predictable paradigm that was broken with the introduction of diagnostic MR imaging. MR imaging provides soft tissue contrast in a literally unprecedented manner. However, much of the science underlying the MR imaging process is foreign and entirely non-intuitive to many radiologists. Indeed, the name of our profession itself - radiology - underscores its dependence upon x-rays and ionizing radiation-based imaging - and not one based on magnetic fields.

MR imaging introduces several significant and quite nonintuitive changes into the ionizing radiation–based safety risk assessment model described above. With MR imaging, we are no longer dealing with a single energy source; rather, multiple energy sources are required to produce these powerfully diagnostic images. Furthermore, each of these energy sources is associated with its own risk or set of risks, and these differ from those of each of the other energy sources used in diagnostic MR imaging studies. In addition, the spatial distribution of these energy sources is not only heterogeneous, but each of the various fields or energies used in the MR imaging process has its own unique spatial distribution pattern. To make matters worse, the *temporal* distribution of these energy sources also differs among the various energies and fields used in the MR imaging process. Some are present only during active imaging; others are present even when no imaging is taking place. In fact, some of these energies may be present even when the system is apparently inactive and "off," when no patients are being examined, and the site itself is powered down for the night!

With MR imaging, our comfortable safety model is dramatically modified (**Table 1**). To safely perform MR imaging on our patients, we have to learn an entirely new paradigm and must be able to logically apply that new algorithm and understanding to patient and device safety evaluations. That has proven to be both daunting and frustratingly nonintuitive for most of its practitioners.

This article focuses on precisely this algorithm. It would require a textbook to provide the details and nuances of each energy, their myriad associated risks, their unique spatial distributions subtleties, and their customized risk mitigation strategies. However, the purpose of this exercise is to provide an outline of the major underlying issues followed by an algorithm that can be successfully applied toward systematically assessing and even pseudo-quantifying the risks associated with MR scanning of patients with implanted devices, implants, and/or foreign bodies.

ENERGIES/FIELDS

Every MR imaging study uses 3 different energies or fields that can be broken down into 4 fields, as follows.

Static Magnetic Field (Bo)

Intrinsic in the clinical MR imaging process is the requirement to magnetize the hydrogen nuclei of the tissues being imaged. This process is accomplished by exposing the patient to a powerful static magnetic field, commonly referred to as the Bo magnetic field. The most commonly used static magnetic field strengths used in clinical MR imaging today are 1.5 T followed by 3 T. This static magnetic field Bo can be thought of as having a "frequency" of zero, because it never changes before, during, or after the patient undergoes their MR imaging study.

Static Magnetic Field Gradient (dB/dx)

As one approaches the MR scanner, the strength of that MR scanner's static magnetic field increases. One could thus map the *spatial rate of change* of the magnetic field that envelopes that MR scanner, where the spatial rate of change of

Table 1
Differences between radiograph/computed tomography- and MR imaging-based risk assessments

Modality	Radiograph/Computed Tomography	MR Imaging
Number of fields and/ or energy sources	1	3 (4)
Associated risks	All associated with ionizing radiation (carcinogenesis, cataractogenesis)	Varied, with unique risks associated with each energy or field used in the MR imaging process
Irradiation pattern	Homogeneous through the anatomy being evaluated	Heterogeneous and homogeneous throughout the anatomy being evaluated, and heterogeneous outside of the volume being evaluated
Potential risk exposure	Only the anatomy/volume being evaluated	Tissue and structures within as well as physically quite distant from the anatomy/volume being evaluated
Temporal associations of potential risks	Only during active imaging	Some are only present during active MR imaging; others are active at all times, whether the system is imaging or even "on" or not

the magnetic field as one gets closer to the scanner increases the closer one gets to the scanner itself. For example, at the entrance to the room containing the MR scanner, with each centimeter one approaches the scanner opening, the magnetic field might get 1 G stronger. However, at close proximities to the MR scanner with each centimeter closer that one gets to the scanner, the magnetic field might measure 1000 G stronger! Thus, the spatial rate of change, or dB/dx, associated with the Bo static magnetic field of that scanner can be mapped out and is stronger in certain locations in the room and In the magnet bore than in other regions. Of course, because the Bo magnetic field is, by definition, static or constant, this spatially changing dB/dx magnetic field gradient is also static and does not change over time, hence, the name fixed spatial magnetic field gradient, or magnetic spatial gradient, or fixed field gradient, or spatial field gradient. One could say that it has a "frequency" of zero, because it never changes, just as the "frequency" of change of the static field Bo is zero.

Time-Varying Magnetic Field (Imaging) Gradients (dB/dt)

Time-varying gradient magnetic fields are used for multiple purposes in MR imaging, but one of their most critical functions is to enable spatial localization of the signals detected in the MR imaging process. These magnetic fields, produced by 3 sets of orthogonally oriented spatially coregistered gradient coils, vary in strength in a fixed manner across 1 axis in space. Thus, when a transverse gradient is activated, it generates a magnetic field that is, for example, stronger on the left of the patient in the scanner bore and weaker on the right of that patient at the same time. Further, the rate at which that magnetic field changes from stronger on the left to weaker on the right is fixed and constant. A magnetic field that changes in this fashion would be referred to as a linear magnetic field gradient. Linear gradient magnetic fields are turned on and off thousands or tens of thousands of times during a typical MR imaging sequence.

Time-Varying Radiofrequency Magnetic Fields (B1)

Time-varying radiofrequency (RF) oscillating magnetic fields are irradiated into the patient's tissues in order to effect resonance with the patient's hydrogen nuclei exposed to that MR scanner's Bo magnetic field. It is this resonance that results in the tissues absorbing some of this RF irradiated energy and becoming "excited," and it is manipulation and ultimate detection of this excited energy and how it returns to its baseline that we detect. Detecting how different tissues uniquely handle this resonantly absorbed energy is one of the most basic methods used in the MR imaging process to differentiate and contrast various tissues from each other. This B1 energy is itself oscillating at millions of times per second, and hence, the name *radiofrequency* (the precise frequency of which is determined by the strength of the Bo magnetic field of that particular MR scanner). Furthermore, this same RF magnetic field is itself transmitted as pulses, and dozens or hundreds of such pulses may be transmitted per second (depending on the precise MR imaging study design). Thus, technically, the RF (B1) energy is an RF oscillating magnetic field B1 that is itself modulated at extremely low-frequency rates.

DESCRIPTION OF ASSOCIATED RISKS

Each of the above 4 energies or fields is associated with its own risk or set of risks. The predominant ones are included in later discussion. Please note that potential biologic risks, such as mutagenicity/carcinogenesis or acoustic noise, are beyond the scope of this article and will not be discussed herein.

Static Magnetic Field (Bo) and Static Field Gradient (dB/dx) Associated Potential Risks

Because the Bo and dB/dx magnetic fields are constant, the risks associated with the Bo and dB/dx magnetic fields are themselves also always present, even when the MR scanner is "off" and not being used for imaging. The main risks associated with a static magnetic field Bo and its associated static field gradient dB/dx include those associated with induced forces on ferromagnetic materials/objects within that field. Such forces include the following:

1. Torque: Ferromagnetic objects in the field with asymmetric aspect ratios experience a force that would tend to align their long axes parallel to the lines of force associated with that field. The stronger the Bo static field to which such a ferromagnetic material/device is exposed, the stronger the torque related forces.
2. Translation: As one first approaches an MR scanner's magnetic field, ferromagnetic objects approaching the MR scanner would experience a pulling force that would translate or "slide" that object toward the magnet opening. This force is itself determined (among other factors) by the strength of the static field Bo at the location where the ferromagnetic object is found as well as the static field gradient dB/dx across the ferromagnetic object at that position in space. In general, the stronger the static magnetic field Bo (until magnetic saturation is achieved in the ferromagnetic material/object) and the greater the spatial fixed gradient (dB/dx) across the object, the stronger the displacement translational, or "missile effect," related forces attempting to displace the object toward the higher field strength (greater dB/dx) locations.
3. Device modification/alteration: Incapacitation or alteration of the function of a device may result from exposure of that device to strong static magnetic fields Bo and/or static magnetic field gradients dB/dx. This is another risk associated with Bo and dB/dx distinct from that of physical harm from torque or translational forces experienced by ferromagnetic materials exposed to these fields.
4. Lenz's forces: Even if material is NON-ferromagnetic, electrically conductive material moved through static field gradients can result in induced voltages and currents within the moved material. These in turn can secondarily generate magnetic fields that oppose the original motion vector. Thus, there are grossly detectable forces on electrically conductive materials even if they are nonferromagnetic, such as aluminum, that are moved through the static magnetic fields associated with an MR scanner. The more rapid the movement, the greater the strength of these induced Lenz's forces. Thus, rapid motion of certain devices or implants in the immediate vicinity of the entrance to the MR scanner can result in grossly detectable forces on almost any metal devices, implants, materials, or foreign bodies. These may vary from barely perceptible induced forces to overt dislodgement of the implant.

Imaging Gradients (dB/dt) Associated Potential Risks

There are several risks associated with time-varying gradient magnetic fields dB/dt. For example, the auditory sounds or noises associated with the MR imaging process can be sufficiently strong to result in hearing loss. However, as the focus of this article is implant safety, these will not be further elaborated upon here. Furthermore, although heating of implants from exposure to sufficiently strong and prolonged dB/dt is possible, at today's exposure values these are typically minor levels of heating and are not generally a major safety issue associated with dB/dt energies.

The primary risk associated with dB/dt energies is that of inducing neuroexcitation of nerves exposed to sufficiently strong/long time-varying dB/dt, or imaging gradients. Such excitation would be expected to be accompanied by excitation of whatever was at the distal end of the excited nerve. If it would be a muscle, then twitching of that muscle might result. If the heart would be found at the end of that nerve, such neuromuscular excitation or "twitching" would be referred to as an arrhythmia. The likelihood of such arrhythmogenesis would be greatly potentiated if a wire or lead would be in the volume exposed to time-varying dB/dt energies, focusing those induced electrical fields at the tip of that wire or lead where the heart muscle is found.

Radiofrequency (B1) Associated Potential Risks

By far, the single major risk associated with tissues exposed to irradiated RF energies is that of power deposition or heating. Diffuse patient heating and core hyperthermia is one such potential risk, but once again, because this article deals with implant safety, that will not be further dealt with herein. Focal heating, however, can also result from RF irradiation, and that can be of sufficient magnitude to result in thermal injury/burns. It is important, however, to understand that it is not the transmitted time-varying oscillating B1 magnetic fields that heat the tissue. Rather, these transmitted B1 magnetic fields in turn induce time-varying electrical (E) fields, and it is these E-fields that can produce focal energy/heat deposition sufficient to result in thermal injury or burns. Accurately assessing implant/device safety in MR environments absolutely requires a recognition of the above, because this is what is responsible for the potential to induce burns at locations that might be physically quite remote from the B1 irradiated volume. In this regard, wires or leads exposed even in part to the transmitted RF (B1) energies may be uniquely efficient in focusing or concentrating these secondarily induced electrical fields at and just beyond the tip of these leads, an ideal setup for an RF-induced thermal injury or burn.

SPATIAL LOCATION OF ENERGIES/FIELDS AND, THEREFORE, RISKS
Static Field (Bo) Associated Potential Risks: Torque

The static magnetic field of MR scanners is always homogeneous and near its maximum strength in the region in which MR imaging is performed. Therefore, torque-related forces are always strong or near maximal at the center of the MR scanner where imaging is performed.

The spatial distribution of the Bo static field for a typical 1.5-T superconductive MR scanner is depicted in **Fig. 1**.

Static Field Gradient (dB/dx) Associated Potential Risks: Translational Forces, Lenz's Forces, Device Function Alteration/ Incapacitation

The homogeneity of the magnetic field in the volume in which MR imaging is performed means that the spatial field gradient (dB/dx) is at or near zero in the center of the scanner. Therefore, translational or missile-effect forces are ironically *weakest* in the center of the MR scanner. However, these forces reach maximal values as one approaches the physical ends/borders of the magnet coils of the MR scanner (regardless of whether the field is horizontal or vertical). For cylindrical bore configuration superconductive MR scanners, this means that the greatest translational forces are near the entrance to (and exit from) the bore, radially peripherally at the plastic faceplate of the scanner itself. For vertical field systems, the greatest dB/dx and therefore vertically oriented translational forces are typically also located near the radial outer edges of the scanner "plates" and are least and weakest in the (radial) center of the scanner. The spatial distribution of the dB/dx static magnetic field gradient for a typical 1.5-T superconductive MR scanner is depicted in **Fig. 2**.

Imaging Gradient (dB/dt) Associated Potential Risks: Neuromuscular Excitation

The shape of the 3 orthogonal imaging gradients is such that they tend to increase as we approach the left-right, anteroposterior, and superoinferior margins of the gradient coils themselves. Similar to a see-saw in a child's playground, the greatest change per unit time is at the ends of the produced magnetic field gradient/see-saw, and the smallest change per unit time is at its center. The center of the 3 gradient coils is physically coregistered to the center of the Bo magnetic field. Thus, the smallest dB/dt is at the center of the scanner, right where we positioned whatever anatomy of interest it is that we are imaging. At the radial periphery of the scanner are the strongest X (transverse) and Y (anteroposterior) gradients, and (depending on the design of the gradient coils) roughly 35 cm superior and 35 cm inferior to the center of the scanner is where the superoinferior gradient dB/dt maxes out. Thus, implanted or abandoned wires or leads in these positions would have the greatest induced voltages and currents from time-varying gradient dB/dt magnetic field, and therefore, the greatest potential for neuromuscular excitation is found at these locations.

Note that direct neuromuscular excitation of peripheral nerves, or peripheral nerve stimulation (PNS), is what is targeted by regulatory agencies.

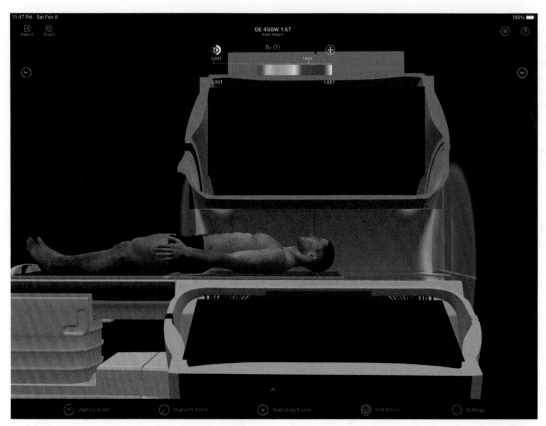

Fig. 1. Figs. 1–4 are 3-dimensional depictions of (for illustration purposes) a GE Healthcare 1.5-T 450-W MR scanner. For teaching purposes, the right side of the scanner has been rendered transparent so that the energies/fields can be depicted as they are distributed 3 dimensionally throughout the MR scanner bore and room. The strength and spatial distribution of the static magnetic field Bo are depicted. (*Courtesy of* Dr Kanal, created using the MagnetVision app that he created, Advanced Magnetic Analytics, LLC.)

PNS itself is not typically harmful per se. However, PNS is achieved at lower levels of neurostimulation than is cardiac muscle stimulation. Therefore, if we do not see/experience PNS, we would not expect to be near cardiac stimulation thresholds. All this changes, however, if there is a wire or lead in the heart. This wire or lead has the potential to temporally and spatially focus induced electrical fields at the tip of the lead and can thus markedly potentiate arrhythmogenesis. Consider the situation of an abandoned cardiac lead where at least part of this lead is exposed to the dB/dt magnetic fields. The study may be centered on the L4 vertebral body for a lumbar spine study, but 35 cm or so superior to this location an abandoned lead in the heart may be exposed to maximal (superoinferior) dB/dt magnetic fields. Such a patient might therefore be exposed to significant arrhythmogenic stimulation despite the fact that the study in question is centered on anatomy that is physically remote from the heart and its abandoned lead.

The spatial distributions of the dB/dt time-varying imaging gradient magnetic fields for a typical 1.5-T superconductive MR scanner are depicted in **Fig. 3**.

Radiofrequency (B1) Associated Potential Risks: Thermal Injury/Burns

The transmitted RF (B1) oscillating magnetic fields induce time-varying electric (E) fields in electrically conductive materials, such as patient tissue. At locations of greater B1 magnitudes, there is the potential for greater induced E fields. B1 magnetic field maps associated with transmitting RF coils are dependent on many factors, including the shape and design of the transmitting RF coil. However, for typical birdcage coil designs, the greatest B1 fields are generally located radially nearest the physical edges of the coil itself, as well as at the superoinferior borders of the transmitting RF coil. There can be extremely rapid decay of B1 amplitude as one leaves the edges of the transmitting

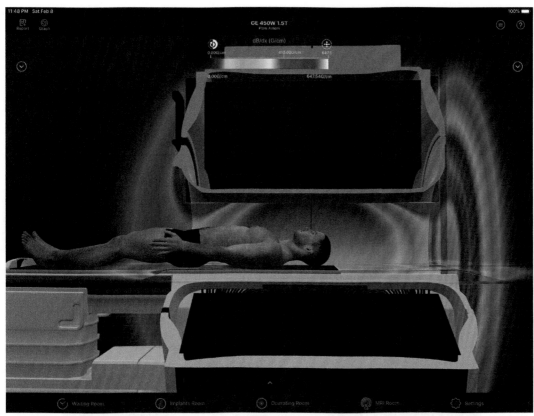

Fig. 2. The strength and spatial distribution of the static/fixed spatial magnetic field gradient dB/dx. Notice that in the homogeneous static magnetic field at the center of the MR scanner, the strength of the dB/dx and therefore potential translational forces on ferromagnetic materials and objects are minimal. The greatest translational forces scale with the dB/dx of this magnet, which maximizes near the radial extremes/borders at the entrance (and exit) to the MR scanner bore. (*Courtesy of* Dr Kanal, created using the MagnetVision app that he created, Advanced Magnetic Analytics, LLC.)

RF coil and heads toward the radial center of the coil. Indeed, the designs are typically such that the central volume of transmitting RF coils has moderately homogeneous B1 fields, but are quite heterogeneous and significantly higher amplitudes at the extreme radial periphery of the coils. Recall, however, that it is not the B1 fields that are responsible for focal thermal injury/burns, but rather the secondarily induced e-fields. Therefore, the greatest induced e-fields tend to be at the radial periphery of these birdcage transmitting RF coils. However, once again, there is a significant exception to this rule: Should there be an electrically conductive tissue pathway, device, object, or foreign body, and especially, if there is a wire, that is exposed even in part to the transmitted B1 fields, these can be exceptionally efficient at concentrating secondarily induced e-fields at the tip of the wire or lead. Such tissue heating just distal to the lead tip could result *even if the tip of that wire is physically quite removed or distant*

from the volume that underwent primary RF (B1) irradiation!

The spatial distribution of the transmitted time-varying oscillating RF (B1) magnetic fields for a typical 1.5-T superconductive MR scanner's body coil is depicted in **Fig. 4**.

STANDARDIZING THE APPROACH TO MR SAFETY ASSESSMENT FOR PATIENTS WITH IMPLANTS, DEVICES, AND FOREIGN BODIES

It is known that there may be very small risks associated with computed tomographic (CT) scanning of some models of active implanted cardiac devices.[1] Assume a pacemaker patient needs a head CT study. In assessing the risks of proceeding, the provided Food and Drug Administration guidance is quite straightforward: "The probability of x-ray electromagnetic interference is lower when radiation dose and particularly the radiation dose rate are reduced.

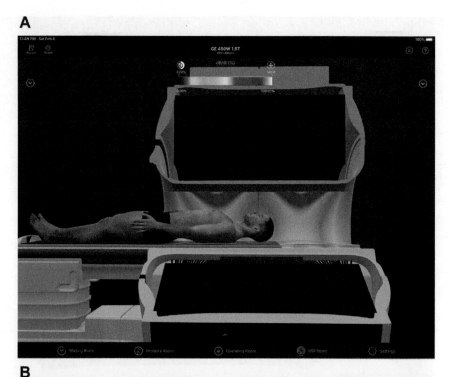

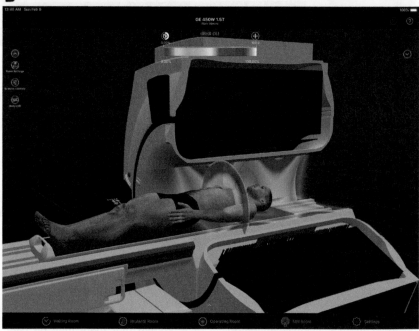

Fig. 3. (*A*) The strength and spatial distribution of the time-varying imaging gradient magnetic fields dB/dt. Note that when centered on the pituitary gland/brain the greatest dB/dt forces are over the chest of this patient, right where a cardiac pacemaker might be positioned. (*B*) The 3-dimensional nature of the 3 orthogonally oriented gradient magnetic fields, which increase in strength as the radial and superoinferior distance from center increases, and approaching the physical margins of the 3 gradient coils. (*Courtesy of* Dr Kanal, created using the MagnetVision app that he created, Advanced Magnetic Analytics, LLC.)

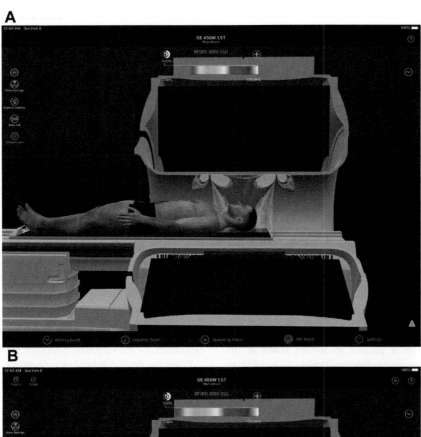

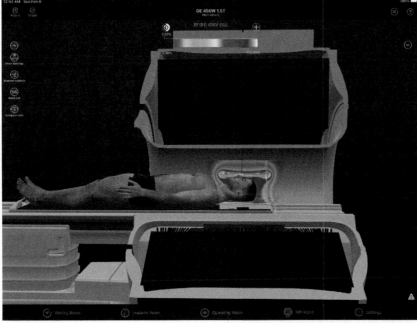

Fig. 4. (*A*) The spatial distribution of the transmitted RF (B1) oscillating magnetic fields with the body coil of this scanner being used as the RF transmitter hardware. (*B*) Note how the transmitted RF fields cover a smaller volume when a transmit-receive head coil is used for RF transmission in this same scanner. (*Courtesy of* Dr Kanal, created using the MagnetVision app that he created, Advanced Magnetic Analytics, LLC.)

Interference can be completely avoided when the implantable device is outside of the primary x-ray beam of the CT scanner." In other words, if you do not irradiate the device, there is no increased risk from CT scanning of such devices! As a famous self-defense instructor once taught, the best defense against a blow is to not be there when it lands.

Note that a risk was detected, and a means was implemented, to mitigate this risk to acceptable levels, thus permitting one to proceed with the requested head CT study on this pacemaker patient. The general algorithm of risk assessment has always been to (a) identify the potential risk(s) from the energy to be used for the requested examination; (b) quantify the risk to the patient/fetus/device for the requested study; then (c) either accept the potential benefit as being substantially greater than the perceived risk OR find a way to mitigate the potential risk back down to acceptably low levels (such as by ensuring that the fetus or implant were not exposed to the energy in question), and safely proceeded with the requested examination. Alternatively, cancel the examination if the potential risk is greater than the potential benefit of the study.

We have seen that MR imaging does not use one, but rather several, energy sources, each with its own associated potential risks and spatial and temporal distributions. Thus, to determine the safety of proceeding with a requested MR imaging examination on a patient in whom there is an implanted device or foreign body, it would be logical to follow the model that we have successfully used above. However, a few modifications are needed to accommodate the fact that multiple energy sources are used in MR imaging:

1. Identify the energy source and its associated potential risks;
2. Assess if the implant/foreign body would be exposed to this energy and therefore its associated risks;
3. Determine if these risks are acceptably low are not;
4. If the risks are at a concerning level, determine if any actions might be undertaken to mitigate those risks to acceptably low levels (relative to the potential benefit of proceeding with the examination in that same patient);
5. Repeat steps 1 to 3 for each of the energy sources used in the MR imaging process;
6. Repeat steps 1 to 5 for each implant, device, and/or foreign body in that patient.

If at any time through this process the potential risks significantly exceed the potential benefit of proceeding with the requested MR imaging study and cannot be mitigated, the examination should likely be canceled. If there are no or low risks from a given energy, and/or if risks might be present but can be successfully mitigated by some interventions effected by the user/operator, proceed with evaluation of the next energy to be used. This process is then repeated until all energies are considered, and no significant risks remain. This entire process is then repeated for all implants, devices, and/or foreign bodies in the patient. If no significant risks remain for any of the energies for any of the implants/foreign bodies in that patient, the potential benefit would likely exceed the low detected cumulative risks of proceeding.

Example 1

A 208 cm 32-year-old male semiprofessional basketball star with an abandoned left subclavian vein to inferior vena cava cardiac lead is requested to undergo an elective 1.5-T MR imaging examination of his right knee for a possible medial meniscal tear. Application of the above described standardized approach to risk assessment would produce the following (assessment questions in *italics*, responses in **bold**):

Energy #1: **Static field Bo.**
Associated risks: **Torque and translation.**
Is the device significantly exposed to this energy/field for the requested study? **Yes.**
Does the device exhibit significant ferromagnetic properties? **No; therefore, no significant associated torque (or translation) risk.**
Risk assessment for this energy: LOW.
Energy #2: **Static field gradient dB/dx.**
Associated risks: **Translation, Lenz's forces.**
Is the device significantly exposed to this energy/field for the requested study? **Yes.**
Does the device exhibit significant ferromagnetic properties? **No; therefore, no significant associated translational risk.**
Is the device electrically conductive? **Yes; therefore, there are potential Lenz's (displacement) forces.**
Can steps be taken to mitigate Lenz's forces? **Yes, move patient slowly through dB/dx fields.**
Risk assessment for this energy: LOW.
Energy #3: **Imaging gradients dB/dt.**
Associated risks: **Neuromuscular excitation/arrhythmogenesis.**
Is the device significantly exposed to this energy/field for the requested study? Recognizing the physical distribution of the dB/dt gradient fields relative to this implant in this patient positioned and centered as they will be for this study, **no, not for the requested study/patient dimensions and positioning; therefore, very low risk of arrhythmogenesis.**
Risk assessment for this energy: LOW.
Energy #4: **Transmitted RF (B1)**
Associated risks: **Thermal injury/burns.**
Is the device significantly exposed to this energy/field for the requested study? **No, not if a**

local transmit/receive extremity coil is used for RF transmission for the requested study/patient positioning; therefore, very low risk of thermal injury/burns.

Risk assessment for this energy: LOW.

Thus, it would seem that for the requested study, for this particular patient, for this particular study requested, for this particular device/implant/foreign body, for the specific MR hardware to be used, the potential risk of proceeding may be quite low.

Example 2

A 173 cm 94-year-old male patient with a suspected ferromagnetic jagged 13-mm foreign body (shrapnel injury from World War II) in the right chest just lateral to the right pulmonary hilum is requested to undergo a 1.5-T MR imaging examination of the lumbar spine for severe low back pain and a left L5 radiculopathy. Application of the above described standardized approach to risk assessment would produce the following:

Energy #1: **Static field Bo.**

Associated risks: **Torque and translation.**

Is the device significantly exposed to this energy/field for the requested study? **Yes.**

Does the device exhibit significant ferromagnetic properties? **Presumed YES; therefore, significant presumed associated torque (and translation) risk.**

Can steps be taken to mitigate torque forces? **NO.**

Torque risk assessment for this energy: HIGH.

Energy #2: **Static field gradient dB/dx.**

Associated risks: **Translation, Lenz's forces.**

Is the device significantly exposed to this energy/field for the requested study? **Yes.**

Does the device exhibit significant ferromagnetic properties? **Yes; therefore, significant presumed associated translational risk.**

Can steps be taken to mitigate torque forces? **NO.**

Is the device electrically conductive? **Yes; therefore, there are potential Lenz's (displacement) forces.**

Can steps be taken to mitigate Lenz's forces? **Yes, move patient slowly through dB/dx fields.**

(Translational) Risk assessment for this energy: HIGH.

Energy #3: **Imaging gradients dB/dt.**

Associated risks: **Neuromuscular excitation/arrhythmogenesis.**

Is the device significantly exposed to this energy/field for the requested study? **Yes, but short electrical length and position in right mid chest**

lateral to the right pulmonary hilum and not in/contiguous with the heart reduce risk for arrhythmogenesis.

Risk assessment for this energy: LOW.

Energy #4: **Transmitted RF (B1)**

Associated risks: **Thermal injury/burns.**

Is the device significantly exposed to this energy/field for the requested study? **Yes, but short electrical length and central position in the chest/bore significantly decrease risk of thermal injury/burns.**

Risk assessment for this energy: LOW.

For this requested study, for this particular patient, for this device/implant/foreign body, for the specific MR hardware to be used, the potential risk of proceeding may be quite high from torque/translation of a jagged metallic piece of World War II shrapnel next to major pulmonary vasculature and the lung parenchyma itself. One might well consider canceling the requested study as the potential life-threatening risk of proceeding would far exceed the potential diagnostic benefit of a lumbar spine MR imaging for radiculopathy.

We can see how changing ANY of these clinical parameters (eg, requested study is a head or cervical spine MR imaging instead of knee, or different implant, or different patient/body habitus) requires us to start from scratch and perform a new safety assessment, because the answers and therefore risk quantification levels are specific to each presenting clinical situation.

SUMMARY

MR imaging is unique in that multiple energy sources are used to generate every MR study. The relative spatial distributions of these energies and their associated risks are unique to each energy/field. We can standardize our process of attempting to assess and pseudo-quantify the risks associated with MR imaging in patients with devices and/or foreign bodies by

1. Evaluating the potential risks of proceeding with the requested MR imaging study for each MR imaging energy/field for that implant/device/foreign body;
2. Attempting to mitigate any detected risks that might be present for any of the MR imaging energies/fields relative to that implant/foreign body;
3. Repeating this process for each implant, device, and/or foreign body in our patient and assessing final cumulative risks of proceeding with the requested MR imaging study.

By comparing the potential benefit against the final cumulative risks of proceeding with the requested MR imaging study, we will be able to provide the patient with an informed and scientifically sound benefit-risk ratio about the safety of that particular requested MR imaging study, in that patient, on that MR scanner hardware.

ACKNOWLEDGMENTS

Dr. Kanal is the designer, creator, and owner of MagnetVision™, the MR safety software simulator used to generate the illustrations used throughout this manuscript.

DISCLOSURE

The authors have nothing to disclose.

REFERENCE

1. Effects of X-ray irradiation from CT imaging on pacemakers and implantable cardioverter defibrillators (ICD)–literature review. Available at: https://www.fda.gov/radiation-emitting-products/electromagnetic-compatability-emc/effects-x-ray-irradiation-ct-imaging-pacemakers-and-implantable-cardioverter-defibrillators-icd. Accessed February 9, 2020.

FURTHER READINGS

Baker KB, Tkach JA, Nyenhuis JA, Phillips M, Shellock FG, Gonzalez-Martinez J, Rezai AR. Evaluation of specific absorption rate as a dosimeter of MRI-related implant heating. J Magn Reson Imaging 2004;20:315–20.

Delfino JG, Krainak DM, Flesher SA. MRI-related FDA adverse event reports: a 10-yr review. Med Phys 2019;46(12):5562–71.

Dempsey MF, Condon B, Hadley DM. Investigation of the factors responsible for burns during MRI. J Magn Reson Imaging 2001;13:627–31.

Konings MK, Bartels LW, Smits HFM, Bakker CJG. Heating around intravascular guidewires by resonating RF waves. J Magn Reson Imaging 2000;12:79–85.

Mattei E, Triventi M, Calcagnini G, Censi F, Kainz W, Mendoza G, Bassen HI, Bartolini P. Complexity of MRI induced heating on metallic leads: experimental measurements of 373 configurations. Biomed Eng Online 2008;7(11):1–16.

Nyenhuis JA, Park S-M, Kamondetdacha R, Ajad A, Shellock FG, Rezai AE. MRI and implanted medical devices; basic interactions with an emphasis on heating. IEEE Trans Device Mater Reliab 2005;5(3):467–80.

Panych LP, Madore B. The physics of MRI safety. J Magn Reson Imaging 2018;47:28–43.

Panych LP, Kimbrell VK, Mukundan S, Madore B. Relative magnetic force measures and their potential role in MRI safety practice. J Magn Reson Imaging 2020;51:1260–71.

Schaefer DJ, Bourland JD, Nyenhuis JA. Review of patient safety in time varying gradient fields. J Magn Reson Imaging 2000;12:20–9.

Yamazaki M, Yamada E, Kudou S, Higashida M. Study of a temperature rise in RF irradiation during MR imaging: measurements of local temperature using a loop phantom. Japan J Radiol Technol 2005;61(8):1125–32.

MR Safety
Active Implanted Electronic Devices

Robert E. Watson Jr, MD, PhD*, Heidi A. Edmonson, PhD

KEYWORDS

- Electronic implanted devices • MR safety • Cardiac implanted electronic devices
- Neurostimulation systems • Deep brain stimulator • Cochlear implant

KEY POINTS

- Accurate identification of the make and model of any implanted device is essential to ensure the most current conditions for safe MR scanning are used.
- Delaying a diagnosis by denying a clinically warranted scan in the presence of an MR conditional device can harm a patient.
- Coordination of the MR medical director for MR safety, MR safety officer, and MR safety expert facilitates safe scanning.
- An institutional program with radiology and cardiology personnel can allow scanning patients with MR nonconditional cardiac implanted electronic devices.
- Continuing education about implanted devices is essential for optimal patient care. Screening of patients must not fall prey to satisfied search; patients may have more than 1 implanted device.

INTRODUCTION

The variety of active implanted medical devices (AIMD) available for treatment of multiple conditions continues to increase at a rapid rate. These devices are typically implanted to address significant clinical conditions that are likely to require advanced imaging, including MR imaging. They are defined as AIMDs because they contain an energy source such as a battery, or have the ability to be inductively coupled.[1] Such electronic implants contain metallic components, which by definition in ASTM F2503, can be considered only MR conditional or MR unsafe. Any metallic components exclude a device from being considered MR safe.[2] Manufacturers are increasingly aware of the need for patients with devices to require the diagnostic power of MR imaging, and design and testing for the MR environment is becoming common practice as novel implanted devices are developed.

Accurate knowledge of the make and model of any AIMD is of crucial importance, with severe risks if there is failure to identify an AIMD in a patient

undergoing MR imaging. There is a well-documented case in which a patient with an unknown deep brain stimulator suffered radiofrequency (RF)-related burns to the thalami.[3] Undisclosed cardiac pacemakers have been associated with patient deaths. The Emergency Care Research Institute foundation (ECRI) has deemed incomplete AIMD information in MR imaging patients as 1 of the top 10 patient safety risks in 2020.[4] Sound screening processes are essential, and patients and their medical providers should be queried at the time of MR imaging ordering about the presence of implants. In addition, electronic medical records are increasingly incorporating "implanted devices" modules that archive important device-specific information.[5] This information can help with scheduling the patient to the proper MR scanner, ensure the availability of proper equipment such physiologic monitors or designated RF coils, and appropriate personnel (MR safety officers, specifically trained technologists, MR physicists, AIMD programming staff, etc). This device-specific information should be reconciled when the patient reports for MR imaging. Frequently, patients will

Department of Radiology, Mayo Clinic, 200 First Street Southwest, Rochester, MN 55905, USA
* Corresponding author.
E-mail address: watson.robert16@mayo.edu

Magn Reson Imaging Clin N Am 28 (2020) 549–558
https://doi.org/10.1016/j.mric.2020.08.001
1064-9689/20/© 2020 Elsevier Inc. All rights reserved.

mri.theclinics.com

have cards that identify their particular implants. If the device was implanted at another institution, written surgical records should be obtained for a complete description of implant anatomic location and identification of all implanted AIMD system components. Note, verbal relaying of important device-specific information over the telephone should not be permissible owing to potential errors in conveying the information. Similarly, blanket statements purporting to ensure that all implants are MR compatible is unacceptable; MR-compatible terminology was identified to generate confusion and was removed from MR labeling standards with the 2005 release of ASTM F2503.[6] As part of the screening process at the MR facility, ferromagnetic detection equipment can assist in identifying some implanted devices.[7,8]

With positive identification of the device-specific make, model, and anatomic location of the AIMD, several sources exist to identify whether a device is MR unsafe or MR conditional, with associated conditions. These include MRISafety.com, MagResource, the Global Unique Device Identification Database, and the device manufacturer's web sites and field representatives. The US Food and Drug Administration (FDA) oversees the Global Unique Device Identification Database which is a compilation of every device with a unique device identifier. With the unique device identifier number, the Global Unique Device Identification Database web site provides the manufacturer, name of the device, and some MR safety information as to whether the device is MR conditional or MR unsafe. Other sources can then be consulted regarding the necessary conditions for safe scanning. The MagnetVision app is designed to help MR safety professionals assess anticipated risks of an implant before an MR imaging examination (see Emanuel Kanal's article, "Standardized Approaches To Mr Safety Assessment Of Patients With Implanted Devices,"in this issue).

SAFETY CHALLENGES OF MR AND SCANNING ACTIVE IMPLANTED ELECTRONIC DEVICES

The MR environment is associated with multiple challenges to safe scanning in patients with AIMDs. Patient safety issues can be related either to induced injury directly from the device as a consequence of exposure to the different fields inherent in the MR environment (eg, heating of leads) or to secondary injury from device malfunction (eg, infusion pump failure to restart; damaged circuitry in a cardiac pacemaker) as a consequence of exposure to the MR environment. A joint working group of technical experts from the surgical implants community and the MR safety community have collaborated to devise a Technical Standard (ISO/TS10974) describing the MR-related risks to a patient with an AIMD and the associated design controls and testing for such implants.[1] These risks and the source of the MR interactions are summarized in **Table 1**.

Implant Movement

Devices with ferromagnetic content are subject to displacement force and torque from magnetic field interactions. Contemporary AIMDs typically contain very little ferromagnetic material, with some still generally associated with batteries. As the patient crosses the spatial magnetic gradient field while entering the bore of the magnet, nonferrous metals are subject to Lenz forces, with the potential for slight displacement of the implanted object. If perceived, this can potentially be alarming to the patient, and the MR staff must be well aware of this possibility to address this concern effectively with the patient. The potential mobility of the device is related to the degree to which it is contained by fibrous scar tissue or surgically fixed in place. The time-varying gradient magnetic field may additionally cause slight vibration of the implanted object owing to Lenz forces. Particularly for devices implanted off the central axis of the

Table 1 Potential implant patient risks	
Risk to Patient	**Testing**
Heat	RF field-induced heating of the AIMD Gradient field-induced device heating
Vibration	Gradient field-induced vibration
Force	B_0-induced force
Torque	B_0-induced torque
Extrinsic electric potential	Gradient field-induced lead voltage
Rectification	RF field-induced rectified lead voltage
Malfunction	B_0-induced device malfunction RF field-induced device malfunction Gradient field-induced device malfunction

© ISO. This material is adapted from ISO/TS 10974:2018, with permission of the American National Standard Institute (ANSI) on behalf of the International Organization for Standradization. All rights reserved.

body or away from the center of the MR image, there is increasing opportunity for vibration owing to time-varying gradient magnetic fields, for which MR-conditional limits are generally specified.

Heating of Device Components

The heating of device components primarily from the RF field is a major concern. Particularly in the context of neural stimulators and cardiac implanted electronic devices, RF-related heating of leads in close proximity to sensitive tissues can potentially produce severe damage.[3] Conductive materials such as leads may act as resonant antennae, locally amplifying the RF energy used for MR image formation. In insulated leads where induced electric fields are not dissipated over the length of the lead, heating is concentrated at the tip. Temperatures of less than 43° C are not associated with long-term damage. At 60° C there is instant protein denaturation and tissue coagulation. Between 44° and 60°, tissue death is time dependent. Particularly in insulated leads, in which the induced current is not dissipated over the length of the lead and is concentrated at the tip, the lead length within the RF field is an important variable because heating is related to resonant frequency, with maximal heating related to one-half wavelength. The 1.5T and 3T MR systems detect the nuclear magnetic resonance signal of ^{1}H nuclei at 64 MHz (wavelength 52 cm, $^1/_2$ wavelength 26 cm) and 128 MHz (wavelength 26 cm, $^1/_2$ wavelength 13 cm) resonance frequency, respectively. The physical length of the implanted lead may not reflect the true length or design of the conductive material within (there may be internal loops or redundancy of conductive elements within the lead), and a resonant condition may still arise in leads of a variety of physical lengths. Geometric positioning of leads, loops in their course, and interactions with the RF-induced electrical fields created within the human body can all influence the tendency to heat. Importantly, the attachment of a lead to a pulse generator can have a large influence on heating at the lead tip, with a possibility for lead tip temperatures being greatly increased when unattached. As a result, scanning when there are abandoned leads, unattached to a pulse generator, may be associated with an increased risk of heating.[9] Other factors that can influence RF-associated current deposition and heat production include the type of transmit coil used and its position relative to the implant. The majority of clinical receiver arrays rely on an integrated body transmit coil for RF excitation, exposing the majority of the body to RF energy. Smaller transmit/receive coils, that both broadcast RF and detect the emitted signal, are also available on certain MR systems for head or extremity imaging. The smaller head or extremity transmit/receive coils typically deposit the majority of RF within the volume of the coil. MR conditions for implantable devices may specify eligible coils and/or acceptable distances away from the RF coil.

It is important to emphasize that MR conditions, particularly related to RF-induced heating, cannot be presumed at different field strengths or for multinuclear (nonproton) imaging, because the frequency and wavelength of the RF pulses are field strength dependent; for example, conditional safety at 3 T at a specific absorption rate level does not imply conditional safety at 1.5T. Induced current and potential hot spots within devices are also a possibility owing to exposure to rapidly switching gradient magnetic fields.

Device Malfunction

Induced currents within the device from RF and gradient fields may interfere with the control electronics and cause the device to improperly function or reset. The main magnetic B_0 field can also interact with some devices, particularly those with moving components. For example, implantable infusion pump motors typically stop as a consequence of exposure to the main magnetic field (see the Implantable Infusion Pump section).

SCANNING OF PATIENTS WITH SPECIFIC ACTIVE IMPLANTED ELECTRONIC DEVICES

Implanted electronic devices include cardiac devices (pacemakers and defibrillators) and neurostimulators (deep brain, auditory brainstem implant, spinal cord, vagal nerve, sacral nerve, hypoglossal nerve, phrenic nerve, peripheral nerve, and auditory nerve/cochlear implants), as well as implantable medication pumps. An exhaustive discussion of each of these is well beyond the scope of this article. Because conditions for scanning change frequently and new devices are constantly becoming available, it is essential that sites ensure that they are operating with the most up-to-date information available. As always, it is essential to recognize that patients may present with multiple implanted devices and to consider the most restrictive MR conditions across all implanted devices.

It is also important to recognize that, within a particular model of AIMD, there may be multiple configurations using various components or lead models. Testing to determine MR conditions is performed on complete systems, and the MR conditions to safely perform an MR examination may have different limits, depending on which components are used for the system. Each component of the implanted system must be carefully identified to ensure the complete system is MR conditional. Some AIMDs may be constructed with components from multiple manufacturers; in general, such systems with components from multiple manufacturers have not been evaluated for MR safety.

Cardiac Implanted Electronic Devices

Historically, the presence of cardiac implanted electronic devices, including pacemakers and implanted defibrillators, was considered an absolute contraindication for MR imaging. The static magnetic field imparted mechanical forces on ferromagnetic components in the device. Most historical cardiac implanted electronic devices (CIED) devices also made use of Reed switches, electrical connectors activated by magnets, and entering a strong magnetic field could change the programming of the device. The RF field had the potential to heat cardiac leads, affect the programming of the device, or cause it to oversense or undersense cardiac arrhythmias. Gradient magnetic fields were of concern owing to the possibility of inducing life-threatening arrhythmias, inducing voltages that interfered with the sensing of cardiac waveforms, and possibly affecting battery life. Combined field effects interactions were also possible.[10]

Today, biomedical engineering advances have led to the availability of a host of CIEDs that have attained MR conditional labeling such that safe scanning is possible, provided that the conditions for scanning are completely adhered to, including proper device programming, adherence to specified parameters of MR scanning, and performing quality patient monitoring. MR-conditional CIED systems have been designed and tested for safe operation across a range of configurations of patients, MR scanners, positions, coils, and image acquisition techniques.

To address the multitude of patients implanted with CIED systems lacking FDA labeling specific to use in an MR environment, many studies of carefully monitored MR imaging performed in patients with contemporary non–MR-conditional CIED systems indicated that these patients as well could undergo MR examinations after a risk–benefit analysis without identified adverse outcomes.[11–16] Although contemporary CIED systems are more technologically advanced than previous generations owing to improved shielding and internal circuitry, without explicit MR safety design, testing, and regulatory approval for MR conditional labeling, these systems are still technically MR unsafe. With the understanding that not identifying adverse outcomes is not the same as proving absolute safety and does not explicitly test all exposure conditions for any specific system,[17–19] processes and procedures have been identified with MR nonconditional CIED systems that permit patients access to MR imaging. Clearly, continued research needs to investigate patient outcomes in this scenario, but in the meantime guidelines have been published detailing best practices when scanning patients with MR nonconditional CIEDs.[20] This approach also has been endorsed by the American College of Radiology Committee on MR Safety.[21]

The essential components of a program in which patients with nonconditional CIEDs are scanned include an institutional protocol with a responsible MRMD and CIED MD; a medical necessity for the MR scan; no fractured or abandoned leads are permitted; CIED evaluation immediately before and after MR imaging and personnel to program the CIED; electrocardiogram and pulse oximetry are monitored throughout; a defibrillator with external pacing capabilities is available (outside zone IV); and advanced cardiac life support-certified personnel in attendance during the examination until the device is reprogrammed after the MR examination. If the patients has an implantable cardioverter defibrillator, the tachycardia detection and therapies are deactivated. Tachycardia therapies rely on an internal transformer to generate the requisite shock. In large magnetic fields, the transformer is unable to achieve the required voltage, and the device continues to attempt to charge, drawing down the battery life. If therapies are not deactivated, the patient may require replacement of the implantable pulse generator or risk being left without tachycardia therapies after the MR examination.

If the patient is not pacemaker dependent, the device is programmed to nonpacing mode (OVO/OOO) or inhibited mode (VVI/DDI) with deactivation of advanced features. If the patient is pacer dependent, personnel with the ability to establish temporary pacing must be immediately available. The CIED is programmed to asynchronous mode with deactivation of advanced features. Particularly in older CIEDs, power on resets can be encountered rarely in MR imaging[22] and this can be particularly concerning when scanning pacemaker-dependent patients. With the adoption of this approach, in the United States, the Centers for Medicare and Medicaid Services permits reimbursement for MR examinations performed in patients with nonconditional CIED systems.

Deep Brain Stimulation Systems

Deep brain stimulation has been used in the treatment of Parkinson's disease, other movement disorders, epilepsy, and some psychiatric conditions (**Fig. 1**). Particularly as electrodes are implanted in vital brain structures, MR-induced heating can have devastating clinical consequences. A patient undergoing MR imaging of the lumbar spine using a body transmit system suffered a significant lesion in the thalamus on the side ipsilateral to the relatively long lead connected with a pulse generator implanted in the abdomen, resulting in a hemiparesis (**Fig. 2**).[3] Whereas cardiac tissue is highly perfused and difficult to thermally injure in the MR environment, neural tissues are extremely sensitive to even modest temperature elevation. MR safety conditions for scanning deep brain stimulation systems have extreme restrictions on RF deposition, often allowing only 3% to 5% of the RF allowed under the normal mode operation of the MR scanner. Newer labeling uses a patient-independent measure of RF, B1 + root mean squared (B1+rms), in recognition that the coupling between the device and RF is more dependent on the incident RF field rather than the patient's absorption of RF within the body. With the thermally sensitive neural tissue within the densely critical deep brain structures, it is essential that the MR conditions for deep brain stimulation are followed in their entirety, after carefully identifying all implanted components of the system. Limiting the assessment of conditions for safe scanning only to those related, for example, to the pulse generator, without appreciating conditions associated with the implanted leads could pose significant patient hazards. For example, for Medtronic (Dublin, Ireland) deep brain stimulation systems, the presence of a pocket adapter near the pulse generator precludes use of the body transmit coil, limiting the examination to transmit/receive coils. The pocket adaptors permit older style leads with low impedance (unsuitable for body transmit coil) to be connected to a more contemporary implantable pulse generator at time of implantable pulse generator update.

Spinal Cord Stimulation Systems

Spinal cord stimulation technology is increasingly providing therapeutic options, particularly for patients suffering from chronic pain syndromes. Multiple manufacturers are marketing spinal cord stimulation systems (**Fig. 3**), with some MR unsafe and others MR conditional, including important conditions related to coil choices, including the necessity of using local transmit/receive coils versus allowing body coil transmit. As with other systems involving a pulse generator and neurostimulation or cardiac leads, the entire system of leads and pulse generator must together determine its MR safety status. An MR-conditional spinal cord stimulation pulse generator attached to MR-nonconditional leads makes the system MR nonconditional. The spinal cord level at which spinal cord stimulation electrodes are placed is variable and depends on the patient's clinical symptoms and the particular anatomic segment needing treatment, the antenna of the lead system is thus variable from patient to patient, posing additional challenges to safe scanning. Some MR-conditional systems are currently available that permit scanning using the body coil transmit

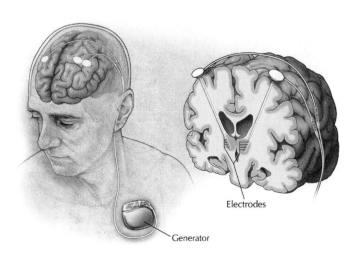

Electrodes

Generator

Fig. 1. Deep brain stimulation system. The system consists of a pulse generator, typically implanted in the infraclavicular region. Leads are tunneled subcutaneously cephalad and over the cranium, where there is attachment to electrodes that are implanted surgically into designated anatomic targets. (Used with permission of Mayo Foundation for Medical Education and Research. All rights reserved.)

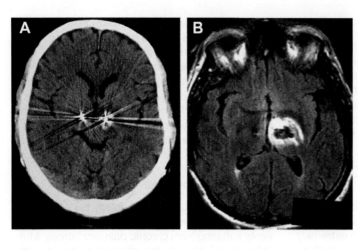

Fig. 2. RF burn centered at the left thalamus, seen in a computed tomography scan (*A*) and T2 fluid-attenuated inversion recovery MR imaging (*B*) images, resulting from a body transmit lumbar spine MR imaging in a patient with a deep brain stimulator. The pulse generator on the patient's left was implanted in the abdomen, apparently permitting excessive RF deposition asymmetrically on this insulated lead, with pronounced heating at the intracranial electrode terminal. (*From* Henderson JM, Tkach J, Phillips M, Baker K, Shellock FG, Rezai AR. Permanent neurological deficit related to magnetic resonance imaging in a patient with implanted deep brain stimulation electrodes for Parkinson's disease: case report. *Neurosurgery.* 2005;57(5):E1063; discussion E1063; with permission.)

have adopted technologies to shield their spinal cord stimulation leads. For example, Medtronic SureScan devices incorporate a braided metallic shield about the leads, functioning as an RF shield, isolating the RF energy from the conductor leads, and dissipating the energy to the adjacent tissues along the length of the lead. RF energy that is conveyed back toward the pulse generator is shunted to its case, where it is dispersed over the soft tissues about it. The Boston Scientific (Marlborough, MA) Precision Montage spinal cord stimulation system with the Avista lead uses a technology termed billabong current suppression in which wires wound about the stimulation lead have short reversed coil sections that suppress induced currents.[23]

It is essential for a number of the MR-conditional systems that the patient brings the AIMD programmer to the MR appointment so that the system can be interrogated, shut off, and/or placed into MR-conditional mode. As with all MR-conditional systems, it is essential that the stated conditions be followed carefully; some, although permitting body coil transmit, are quite restrictive in the

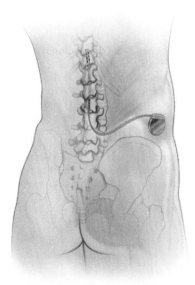

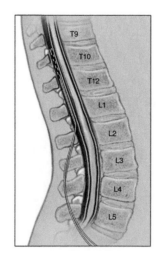

Fig. 3. Spinal cord stimulation system. The system consists of a pulse generator, typically implanted in the subcutaneous posterior soft tissues superior to the iliac bone. Leads are tunneled subcutaneously cephalad and enter the epidural space in the spinal canal. They can be advanced cephalad to the spinal level where there is maximal clinical benefit. Owing to the variability of where the electrodes terminate, it is important to know their position before scanning. Other conditions of scanning, including device programming and impedance checks, are typically performed. (Used with permission of Mayo Foundation for Medical Education and Research. All rights reserved.)

allowable specific absorption rate. Others restrict their use to transmit/receive coils that do not overlap the spinal cord stimulation system, whereas other spinal cord stimulation are considered MR unsafe.

Vagal Nerve Stimulation Systems

Vagal nerve stimulation systems are used primarily to increase seizure control in patients with epilepsy, but are also being used in patients with treatment-resistant depression. The system consists of a pulse generator typically implanted in the infraclavicular region, with a lead terminating about the left vagus nerve in the neck (**Fig. 4**). Vagal nerve stimulation systems from LivaNova, Inc (London, UK), permit scanning at 1.5T and 3T, with certain models restricted to transmit/receive coils, and some newer models allowing use of body transmit; as with other electronic implanted devices, it is essential to carefully identify all components of a patient's implanted system to establish the specific conditions permissible to ensure safe scanning. Before MR imaging, the stimulation parameters are assessed, and device outputs may need to be set to 0 mA. LivaNova vagal nerve stimulation systems fall into either

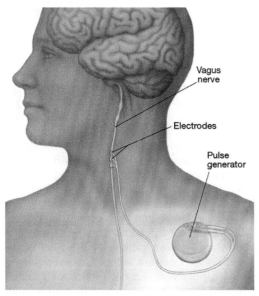

Fig. 4. Vagal nerve stimulation system. The system consists of a pulse generator, typically implanted in the infraclavicular region. Leads are tunneled subcutaneously cephalad and then with deeper dissection, positive and negative helical electrodes are attached to the left vagus nerve, inferior to the cardiac branches.[30] (Used with permission of Mayo Foundation for Medical Education and Research. All rights reserved.)

group A or group B, with group A permitting use of the body coil and scanning outside of the exclusion zone of C7 to L3, and group B permitting use of transmit/receive head or extremity coils outside the exclusion zone of C7 to T8. Not infrequently, vagal nerve stimulation systems are explanted if that patient's epilepsy is not responding to vagal nerve stimulation therapy. Full extraction of the lead from the vagus nerve is a complex procedure with considerable risk to the nerve owing to scarring and tissue alteration about the coiled lead connection region about the nerve. If the nerve is damaged, there can be consequences to speech, cardiac, gastrointestinal, and other functions. In practice, when the vagal nerve stimulation system is explanted, the lead is cut, leaving a short length of lead about the coiled connection with the nerve. It is important to obtain radiographs to determine the length of any retained lead attached to the vagus nerve, because a length of greater than 2 cm precludes the use of body coil transmit.

Sacral Nerve Stimulation Systems

Sacral nerve stimulation has been shown to be efficacious for the treatment of urinary bladder and bowel control. The system consists of a pulse generator typically implanted subcutaneously posteriorly at the upper margin of the buttocks. A lead is implanted adjacent to the sacral nerves (S2, S3, and S4). As of the publication date, MR-conditional sacral nerve stimulator systems do not permit body coil transmit, and are limited to use of transmit/receive head or extremity coils. One manufacturer, Medtronic, has filed a premarket approval supplement with the FDA for approval of its InterStim Micro neurostimulator and also its InterStim SureScan MR imaging leads. InterStim Micro is a rechargeable, implantable sacral neuromodulation device to treat patients affected by overactive bladder, urinary urge incontinence, unobstructed urinary retention, and fecal incontinence. The SureScan leads, which will be used in future implants of the recharge-free InterStim II system and rechargeable InterStim Micro system, are designed to provide full-body 1.5 and 3T-MR conditional labeling, pending approval by the US FDA.

Hypoglossal Nerve Stimulation Systems

A new class of neural stimulators has become available to address obstructive sleep apnea to lessen the need for continuous positive airway pressure. The devices use a lead directed at sensing the onset of a diaphragmatic inspiratory effort, with subsequent stimulation of the hypoglossal nerve, pulling the soft tissues of the tongue anteriorly, and opening the oropharyngeal airway (**Fig. 5**). Some of the devices presently available are MR unsafe, although model 3028 from Inspire, Inc (Golden Valley, MN), is MR conditional. The conditions include that the device is turned off, scanning is at 1.5T in normal operating mode, and the transmit and receive coils of the head or extremities are used that cover no components of the implanted system. As of this writing, no implanted electronic systems using direct stimulation of the phrenic nerve is MR conditional, and are MR unsafe.

Cochlear Implant Systems

Internal components of a cochlear implant system consist of a receiver and stimulator, stimulation electrodes threaded into the cochlea, and an internal magnet that permits coupling with an externally worn transmitter (**Fig. 6**). Devices are associated with specific scanning parameters permitting MR conditional scanning. An ongoing issue with many cochlear implants is the presence of the internal magnet and whether in certain circumstances a risk–benefit analysis and informed consent by the patient favors scanning with the magnet remaining in place. Although an option exists to surgically remove the internal magnet before the MR imaging and replace that after the MR imaging, as with any surgical procedure, there is a risk of infection or other complication. Particularly in patients with cochlear implants who need multiple MR imaging studies, including those with neurofibromatosis type 2 in which growth of

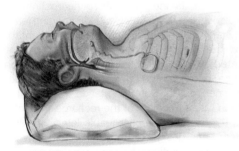

Fig. 5. Hypoglossal nerve stimulation system. The system consists of a pulse generator, typically implanted in the infraclavicular region. The inferior lead is tunneled subcutaneously caudally, and senses onset of an inspiratory effort. The cephalad electrode attaches to hypoglossal nerve branches, and serves to contract the tongue's musculature at appropriate times in the breathing cycle, pulling the tongue anteriorly toward the genu of the mandible, and producing widening of the oropharyngeal airway. (Used with permission of Mayo Foundation for Medical Education and Research. All rights reserved.)

multiple tumors must be periodically assessed, the repeated surgeries for magnet removal can pose a risk. The alternative to magnet removal is to tightly wrap the head in an effort to prevent magnet dislodgement. Head wrapping is associated with patient discomfort and, despite the head wrap, some magnets do dislodge.[24,25] In addition, the presence of the magnet imparts a significant susceptibility artifact, although techniques are available to mitigate these.[26] Increasingly, efforts are underway on the part of cochlear implant manufacturers to address this issue, with 3 manufacturers now each having magnets that self-align to the main magnetic field: MED-EL Synchrony (MED-EL, Innsbruck, Austria; see **Fig. 6**B), Advanced Bionics HiRes Ultra 3D (Advanced Bionics, Los Angeles, CA), and the Nucleus CI600 series (Cochlear Americas, Lone Tree CO), eliminating the need for head wrapping. The reader is referred to an excellent review by Erhardt and colleagues[27] addressing MR safety considerations related to cochlear implants and other intracranial implants. Auditory brainstem implant systems are similar to cochlear implants, with the exception that, owing to anatomic considerations, instead of stimulating the cochlear nerve within the cochlea, electrodes are placed that directly stimulate the cochlear nucleus at the pontomedullary junction at the brainstem. MR conditionally safe scanning can be performed with some of these systems.

Implantable Infusion Pumps

Implantable infusion pumps allow controlled delivery of medications into the subarachnoid space at the spinal canal. The most commonly infused medications are morphine or its derivatives for pain control and baclofen or its derivatives for control of spasticity. While in the MR scanner, the pump may stop owing to the strong magnetic forces, suspending drug infusion. The pump must be assessed after MR imaging, because the gears within the pump motor may temporarily bind and prevent the pump from restarting. This circumstance could potentially lead to opioid withdrawal or baclofen withdrawal syndrome, a serious condition associated with approximately 20% mortality.[28] It is important to note specific conditions for scanning associated with each manufacturers' pump. In particular, although MR conditional, conditions associated with safe scanning of Prometra pumps (Flowonix Medical, Mount Olive Township, NJ) require that the drug reservoir be entirely emptied before patient entry into the scanner. This factor is important, because there is a risk with these devices of

A

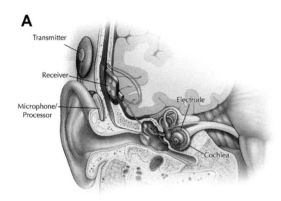

B

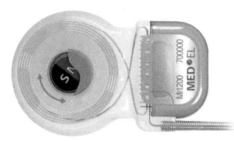

Fig. 6. Cochlear implant. (*A*) A cochlear implant system. It consists of an externally attached auditory microphone processor and transmitter system. This is affixed transcranially to the surgically implanted receiver that delivers stimulation through an electrode implanted into the cochlea to produce sound perception for the patient. The internal/external component attachment is typically accomplished by ferrous elements in the external component that couple with magnets that are an inherent part of the internal implanted device. Newer generations of MR-conditional cochlear implants (*B*) feature rotating magnets that align with the MR main magnetic field, eliminating the substantial torque and attractive forces of earlier generations of these devices. ([*A*] Used with permission of Mayo Foundation for Medical Education and Research. All rights reserved; and [*B*] used with permission: MED-EL. MRI & Cochlear Implants: Superior MRI Safety [blog post]. 2018; Retrieved from https://blog.medel.pro/mri-cochlear-implants-reliability/.)

the drug contents being emptied in an uncontrolled manner during an MR imaging. Safety issues related to implantable infusion pumps in MR imaging were the subject of an FDA alert in 2017.[29]

SUMMARY

The variety and use of active implanted devices continues to proliferate, and their overall benefit to clinical care is unquestioned. Increasingly, manufacturers are engineering MR-conditional systems so that these patients can safely have access to the diagnostic power of MR imaging if MR conditions are carefully met. Diligent pre-MR imaging patient screening is essential to ensure that each and every implant system is identified in its entirety, and conditions for scanning are strictly followed. Severe damage can result with improper scanning conditions, either to the patient's tissue adjacent to the device, or to the continued functionality of the device itself. In the coming years, a host of new innovative devices is likely. With the awareness of the likely concurrent needs of implant recipients to need access to MR imaging, the science behind designing MR conditional systems can be expected to continue to rapidly advance.

DISCLOSURE

The authors declare they have no conflicts of interest or funding to disclose.

REFERENCES

1. ISO/TS 10974:2018. Assessment of the safety of magnetic resonance imaging for patients with an active implantable medical device. 2018. Available at: https://www.iso.org/standard/65055.html. Accessed July 30, 2020.
2. ASTM-F2503 ⟩ Standard practice for marking medical devices and other items for safety in the magnetic resonance environment. Available at: https://www.astm.org/Standards/F2503.htm. Accessed July 30, 2020.
3. Henderson JM, Tkach J, Phillips M, et al. Permanent neurological deficit related to magnetic resonance imaging in a patient with implanted deep brain stimulation electrodes for Parkinson's disease: case report. Neurosurgery 2005;57(5):E1063 [discussion: E1063].
4. Drees J. Top 10 health technology hazards for 2020. Plymouth Meeting. Pennsylvania: ECRI Institute; 2019. Available at: https://www.ecri.org/landing-2020-top-ten-health-technology-hazards. Accessed February 20, 2020.
5. Watson RE, Cradick CM, Epps S, et al. Implementing an electronic health record medical device module-A critical patient safety enhancement. J Am Coll Radiol 2016;13(6):705–8.
6. Shellock FG, Woods TO, Crues JV 3rd. MR labeling information for implants and devices: explanation of terminology. Radiology 2009;253(1):26–30.
7. Shellock FG, Karacozoff AM. Detection of implants and other objects using a ferromagnetic detection system: implications for patient screening before MRI. AJR Am J Roentgenol 2013;201(4):720–5.

8. Watson RE, Walsh SM, Felmlee JP, et al. Augmenting MRI safety screening processes: reliable identification of cardiac implantable electronic devices by a ferromagnetic detector system. J Magn Reson Imaging 2019;49(7):e297–9.

9. Langman DA, Goldberg IB, Finn JP, et al. Pacemaker lead tip heating in abandoned and pacemaker-attached leads at 1.5 Tesla MRI. J Magn Reson Imaging 2011;33(2):426–31.

10. Roguin A, Schwitter J, Vahlhaus C, et al. Magnetic resonance imaging in individuals with cardiovascular implantable electronic devices. Europace 2008; 10(3):336–46.

11. Nazarian S, Hansford R, Rahsepar AA, et al. Safety of magnetic resonance imaging in patients with cardiac devices. N Engl J Med 2017;377(26):2555–64.

12. Russo RJ, Costa HS, Silva PD, et al. Assessing the risks associated with MRI in patients with a pacemaker or defibrillator. N Engl J Med 2017;376(8): 755–64.

13. Rahsepar AA, Zimmerman SL, Hansford R, et al. The Relationship between MRI radiofrequency energy and function of nonconditional implanted cardiac devices: a prospective evaluation. Radiology 2020; 295(2):307–13.

14. Padmanabhan D, Kella DK, Mehta R, et al. Safety of magnetic resonance imaging in patients with legacy pacemakers and defibrillators and abandoned leads. Heart Rhythm 2018;15(2):228–33.

15. Russo RJ. Determining the risks of clinically indicated nonthoracic magnetic resonance imaging at 1.5 T for patients with pacemakers and implantable cardioverter-defibrillators: rationale and design of the MagnaSafe Registry. Am Heart J 2013;165(3): 266–72.

16. Shellock FG. MRI and patients with non-MRI-conditional cardiac devices: further evidence of safety. Radiology 2020;295(2):314–5.

17. Kanal E. Magnetic resonance imaging in cochlear implant recipients: pros and cons. JAMA Otolaryngol Head Neck Surg 2015;141(1):52–3.

18. Woods TO, Delfino JG, Shein MJ. Response to standardized MR terminology and reporting of implants and devices as recommended by the American College of Radiology Subcommittee on MR safety. Radiology 2016;279(3):906–9.

19. Kanal E, Froelich J, Barkovich AJ, et al. Standardized MR terminology and reporting of implants and devices as recommended by the American College of Radiology Subcommittee on MR Safety. Radiology 2015;274(3):866–70.

20. 2017 HRS Expert Consensus Statement on Magnetic Resonance Imaging and Radiation Exposure in Patients with Cardiovascular Implantable Electronic Devices. 2017. Available at: https://www.hrsonline.org/clinical-resources/2017-hrs-expert-consensus-statement-magnetic-resonance-imaging-and-radiation-exposure-patients. Accessed February 20, 2020.

21. Safety ACRCoM, Greenberg TD, Hoff MN, et al. ACR guidance document on MR safe practices: updates and critical information 2019. J Magn Reson Imaging 2020;51(2):331–8.

22. Higgins JV, Sheldon SH, Watson RE Jr, et al. Power-on resets" in cardiac implantable electronic devices during magnetic resonance imaging. Heart Rhythm 2015;12(3):540–4.

23. Gulve A. MRI conditionality across spinal cord stimulation devices: the myths & science 2017. Available at: https://neuronewsinternational.com/mri-conditionality-across-spinal-cord-stimulation-devices-myths-science/. Accessed March 1, 2020.

24. Carlson ML, Neff BA, Link MJ, et al. Magnetic resonance imaging with cochlear implant magnet in place: safety and imaging quality. Otol Neurotol 2015;36(6):965–71.

25. Kim BG, Kim JW, Park JJ, et al. Adverse events and discomfort during magnetic resonance imaging in cochlear implant recipients. JAMA Otolaryngol Head Neck Surg 2015;141(1):45–52.

26. Edmonson HA, Carlson ML, Patton AC, et al. MR imaging and cochlear implants with retained internal magnets: reducing artifacts near highly inhomogeneous magnetic fields. Radiographics 2018;38(1): 94–106.

27. Erhardt JB, Fuhrer E, Gruschke OG, et al. Should patients with brain implants undergo MRI? J Neural Eng 2018;15(4):041002.

28. Mohammed I, Hussain A. Intrathecal baclofen withdrawal syndrome- a life-threatening complication of baclofen pump: a case report. BMC Clin Pharmacol 2004;4:6.

29. Safety concerns with implantable infusion pumps in the magnetic resonance (MR) environment. FDA Safety Communication; 2017. Available at: https://www.fda.gov/medical-devices/safety-communications/safety-concerns-implantable-infusion-pumps-magnetic-resonance-mr-environment-fda-safety. Accessed February 20, 2020.

30. Yang J, Phi JH. The present and future of vagus nerve stimulation. J Korean Neurosurg Soc 2019; 62(3):344–52.

Practical Aspects of MR Imaging Safety Test Methods for MR Conditional Active Implantable Medical Devices

Louai Al-Dayeh, MD, PhD*, Mizan Rahman, PhD, Ross Venook, PhD

KEYWORDS

- AIMD • Implants • Medical devices • MR imaging safety • ISO/TS 10974

KEY POINTS

- MR Conditional implants undergo a wide range of well-developed test methods before receiving FDA approval under the specified conditions of use.
- MR imaging safety test methods for implants are empirical, measurement-based, or numerical modeling-based.
- Conditions of use for MR Conditional devices include a combination of factors that are not easily extrapolated.

INTRODUCTION

Because MR imaging, the unique nonionizing imaging modality, uses three different types of electromagnetic (EM) fields (static, gradient, and radiofrequency [RF]), a patient inside the MR scanner is prone to these fields' interaction with the body. Hence, MR safety standards, such as IEC60601-2-33,[1] dictate limits on field exposure levels and characteristics to reduce patient risks from hazards including RF burns, local and whole-body heating, peripheral nerve stimulation, and cardiac stimulation, among others. Although these risks are well-established, and MR imaging systems have a strong history of safe use, there are many reports of different types of adverse events, including in the Food and Drug Administration (FDA) Manufacturer and User Facility Device Experience database.[2]

If the patient has an implantable medical device, there are added safety concerns for the patient because of the interactions of these fields with the implant. These potential hazards, along with several unfortunate patient injuries related to interactions between MR scanners and implanted devices,[3–8] historically led to appropriately conservative default consideration of implantable devices as being contraindicated for MR imaging. In the mid-1990s, passive medical devices (without any internal power source), such as stents, began to get MR Conditional labeling following guidelines and published safety standards of ASTM International (formerly known as American Society for Testing and Materials)[9,10] and recommended MR imaging safety guidelines per early publications on the subject.[11,12] Because of the many different types of interactions, and potential patient harms, active implantable medical

All authors are employees of Boston Scientific Neuromodulation Corp.
Boston Scientific Neuromodulation, 25155 Rye Canyon Loop, Valencia, CA 91355, USA
* Corresponding author.
E-mail address: louai.aldayeh@bsci.com

Magn Reson Imaging Clin N Am 28 (2020) 559–571
https://doi.org/10.1016/j.mric.2020.07.008
1064-9689/20/© 2020 Elsevier Inc. All rights reserved.

devices (AIMDs; those relying for its functioning on a source of electrical energy or any source of power other than that directly generated by the human body or gravity[13]) continued to be contraindicated at most sites.

Since the first successful MR imaging safety labeling of an implanted Deep Brain Stimulation (DBS) system by Medtronic (Minneapolis, MN) approximately 20 years ago, with significant limitations on applied fields, AIMD manufacturers have come a long way in designing their implants with MR safety in mind and in assessing what conditions of MR scanning (eg, limits of RF and/or gradient) can allow MR imaging without compromising patient safety. The first successful FDA labeling of an MR Conditional pacemaker by Medtronic in 2011[14] marked the beginning of the recent era in which many more patients with implanted devices from manufacturers across the industry now have access to MR imaging through MR Conditional labeling.

What facilitated getting to the current state of MR Conditional devices today is a joint effort that started in 2006 across the MR imaging safety community, including representatives from implanted device manufacturers, scanner manufacturers, and regulatory bodies. Experts in each area formed a joint working group that participated in various technical venues helping to shape and update multiple standards. A major outcome of this effort was publication of an international technical specification (TS), ISO/TS 10974, documenting guidelines on the assessment of MR imaging safety for patients with an AIMD. The first version of this TS published in 2012,[15] and the second updated version published in 2018.[16] The work is ongoing, and the group is updating and transitioning the TS into an international standard, with expected publication in 2021 or 2022.

To have a specific focus, this article mainly addresses AIMDs with extended leads (eg, cardiac leads or neuromodulation leads), that is, an implanted pulse generator (IPG) plus one or more leads (see **Fig. 1** for a representative spinal cord stimulator).

RELEVANT FACTS TO COUNTER MISCONCEPTIONS ABOUT MR IMAGING SAFETY TESTING OF ACTIVE IMPLANTABLE MEDICAL DEVICES

- There are many types of potential patient hazards, which require comprehensive testing. It is not simply about magnetic materials or RF burns.
- Most implants that allow MR imaging scanning are MR Conditional; there is practically

no "MR Safe" active implant. In general, if the implant has metallic components, it is either MR Conditional or MR Unsafe.
- What is MR Conditional is a specific device/ system (specific pulse generator + specific lead) per the device's formal MR imaging safety label conditions listed in its instructions for use/manual.
  - No generalizations of MR safety can be made about any other device/system from the same manufacturer or other manufacturers (eg, lead extensions that are not included in the MR label, and not MR Conditional).
- Mixing and matching a pulse generator from an MR Conditional device/system with leads from another MR Conditional device/system does not make the new combination MR Conditional. There is typically no testing or data available to assess such combinations.
- Fractured leads, abandoned leads, and other damaged or nonfunctional implants are typically not assessed for safety, and their level of risk is unknown.
- There are no strong guidelines on how to safely scan a patient with multiple AIMDs (eg, a pacemaker and a spinal cord stimulator). Even if each system is MR Conditional by itself, the multisystem combination is not in general labeled for MR Conditional safety, because of the lack of testing on such combinations.
- Almost all present safety testing and MR Conditional labeling of implants is for either 1.5-T or 3-T cylindrical bore MR imaging scanners (or both). Open-bore systems, and higher- or lower-field scanners, typically are not included in testing standards or in MR Conditional labels.
- If an MR Conditional device/system is deemed safe in a specific MR field strength (eg, 1.5 T), this has no implication on MR safety of the device within other field strengths (eg, lower B0, such as 1 T, or higher B0, such as 3 T or 7 T). No presumption of safety can be made at any field strength other than the one at which the safety assessment was done, because the RF-dependent properties of the system change significantly (eg, RF wavelength, current deposition on leads, exposure fields in the patient caused by scanner design differences) and could be either more safe or less safe.
- In general, accessories of devices/systems (eg, remote control, charger) are not MR Conditional, and many are MR Unsafe and cannot be brought into Zone 4 (the MR imaging scanner room) of the imaging facility.

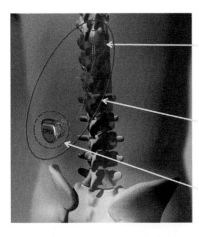

Distal array of Lead
Distal Heating (RF)
Unintended stimulation (RF + GRD)
Lead Injection (RF + GRD)

IPG and Lead System
Vibration (GRD + B_0)
Force/Torque (B_0)

IPG/Proximal Lead
IPG Heating (RF + GRD)
Lead Injection (RF + GRD)
Rectification (RF)
IPG malfunction (B_0 + RF + GRD)

Fig. 1. Illustration of a generic spinal cord stimulator system as an example of AIMD with extended leads. Various potential MR imaging hazards are listed (with reference in parentheses to the causing fields). B0, static field; GRD, time-varying gradient field. Note that understanding the induced fields for an AIMD for RF and time-varying gradients includes surgical implantation variables, such as lead subcutaneous routing and coiling of the lead in the IPG pocket.

MR IMAGING AND ACTIVE IMPLANTABLE MEDICAL DEVICES INTERACTIONS: POTENTIAL SAFETY HAZARDS (PER ISO/TS 10974)

Demonstration of MR Conditional status by implantable device manufacturers (eg, to achieve FDA labeling) involves testing hundreds or thousands of different exposure conditions and modeling many thousands or millions of such potential exposure conditions. This includes exposure in realistic MR imaging scanning environments, benchtop injection testing, and development of appropriate risk assessments though physical experiments and modeling. The quick methods used by some researchers of trying to assess device safety through testing of a handful of configurations of a device within a box of tissue simulating medium (which was common in past decades, and still finds its way into the literature) is simply insufficient. Although it is a helpful first step, or potentially useful In demonstrating hazards, it unfortunately does not meaningfully evaluate safety. This section of the article describes the full range of proper test methods, per established standards, that collectively form the testing package regulatory bodies review for a given MR Conditional device label.

Per ISO/TS 10974:2018[16] the potential safety hazards caused by the MR imaging scanner and AIMD interaction physics are listed in **Table 1**. **Fig. 2** also illustrates these hazards. Each of the three different types of EM fields in a scanner (B0, time-varying gradient, and RF) generate specific interactions and potential safety hazards for patients, as do the different combinations of fields (eg, device vibration is a result of the combination of B0 + time-varying gradient fields).

Most test methods described in various standards do not include explicit acceptance criteria

(eg, how many degrees centigrade of temperature rise is acceptable for electrode heating) because the standards must work for many different types of implants. Because the risk level depends on the nature and location of the implant, and tissues surrounding it, each implant manufacturer must set and justify acceptance criteria for each potential hazard according to their internal risk management procedures, subject to review by regulatory authorities. Typically, this includes using internal company data from a combination of relevant history of safe use, human trials, or animal studies, and accepted literature references. Implant manufacturers are also working on creating vertical standards for a specific type of implants with relevant acceptance criteria for these hazards.

Table 2 includes a more detailed view on one way an AIMD manufacturer might consider and address the wide variety of potential safety hazards and acceptance criteria.

TEST METHODS ADDRESSING POTENTIAL SAFETY HAZARDS CAUSED BY MR IMAGING AND ACTIVE IMPLANTABLE MEDICAL DEVICES INTERACTION: PULSE GENERATOR + LEADS

Evaluation of the AIMD for MR imaging hazards involves benchtop testing, modeling, MR scanners, or a combination of these approaches. One way to categorize these evaluations is whether modeling is a part of the assessment or not (**Table 3**).

B0-Induced Force

A displacement force produced by the static magnetic field (B0) on a device containing magnetic materials has the potential to cause unwanted movement of the implanted device.

Table 1
Potential patient hazards and corresponding test methods

Hazard	Test Method	Clause
Heat	RF field-induced heating of the AIMD	8
	Gradient field-induced device heating	9
Vibration	Gradient field-induced vibration	10
Force	B0-induced force	11
Torque	B0-induced torque	12
Unintended stimulation	Gradient field-induced lead voltage (extrinsic electric potential)	13
	RF field-induced rectified lead voltage	
Malfunction	B0 field-induced device malfunction	14
	RF field-induced device malfunction	15
	Gradient field-induced device malfunction	16
	Combined fields test	17

Each clause of the test method document defines the specific conditions for the testing to ensure proper coverage in the MR imaging environment.

From ISO/TS 10974:2018. Assessment of the safety of magnetic resonance imaging for patients with an active implantable medical device; with permission.

Force exerted on the device is a function of the spatial gradient of B0 (or the product of B0 and the spatial gradient of B0, depending on whether the materials are greater or less than magnetic saturation) and the mass of magnetic material. This established test method is described in ASTM F2052,[17] is measurement-based, and is typically conducted in a scanner.

The concept of testing is to measure the magnetically induced displacement force of the implant where the spatial gradient is greatest (near the opening of the bore) and compare against the gravitational force acting on the device (because all implanted devices are subjected to the force caused by gravity without patient harm). One version of this test is to suspend the device by a thin string at that location and measure the deflection angle; if it deflects less than 45°, its magnetic force is less than that of gravity.

Implants with a displacement force less than the force of gravity are automatically deemed acceptable. If that force is greater, it still could be acceptable with appropriate justification of an appropriate acceptance criterion to maintain patient safety.

For most AIMDs with extended leads, with the main magnetic components implanted subcutaneously and far from vulnerable structures, B0-induced force is not considered a high-risk hazard. There is real potential for concern if the device is in a sensitive physiologic location (eg, brain aneurysm clip).

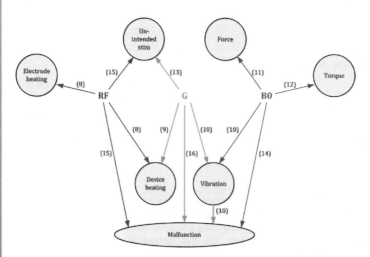

Fig. 2. Relationship between MR imaging scanner output fields RF, gradient (G), static (B0), and hazards (ISO/TS 10974 test method clause numbers in parentheses). (*From* ISO/TS 10974:2018. Assessment of the safety of magnetic resonance imaging for patients with an active implantable medical device; with permission.)

Table 2
Example list of MR imaging–AIMD safety hazards, each of which generates requirements that an AIMD manufacturer must assess with appropriate test methods and rationale

Requirement	10,974 Clause	Details of Meeting Requirement	Rationale/Source
RF-induced lead heating patient harm limit	8	When exposed to RF fields, heating of the lead shall not exceed XX CEM 43°C[21]	ISO/TS 10974 Tissues around lead heating acceptance criteria MR imaging environment exposure durations, levels
Device (IPG) heating patient harm limit: Gradient-induced RF-induced	8 9	When exposed to combined RF and gradient fields, the thermal exposure of tissue surrounding the pocket shall not exceed XX CEM 43°C	ISO/TS 10974 Tissues around stimulator heating acceptance criteria MR imaging environment exposure durations, levels MR imaging EMC acceptance criterion
Gradient-induced vibration patient harm limit	10	When exposed to combined static and gradient fields, the pressure exerted by implanted IPG or leads on the tissue shall not exceed XX psi	ISO/TS 10974 MR imaging vibration tissue damage acceptance criteria MR imaging environment exposure durations, levels
B0-induced force patient harm limit	11	When exposed to static field: Translational force on the IPG shall not exceed XX N Translational force on any implantable system components shall not exceed the weight of the component	ASTM F2052 MR imaging force torque acceptance criterion MR imaging environment exposure durations, levels
B0-induced torque patient harm limit	12	When exposed to static field: Torque on the IPG shall not exceed XX Nm Torque on all implanted system components shall not exceed the weight times the length of the longest side of the component	ASTM F2213 MR imaging force torque acceptance criterion MR imaging environment exposure durations, levels

(continued on next page)

Table 2
(continued)

Requirement	10,974 Clause	Details of Meeting Requirement	Rationale/Source
Electric potential patient harm limit Gradient-induced, extrinsic RF-induced and RF rectification	13 15	When exposed to combined RF and gradient fields: The current conducted by the IPG shall not exceed a pulse charge limit of XX µC in each electrode Amplitude of the current pulse shall not exceed XX µA in IPG stimulation-off condition Amplitude of the current pulse shall be within specified tolerances in IPG stimulation-on condition	ISO/TS 10974 MR imaging environment exposure durations, levels
RF-induced device malfunction limit	15	When exposed to RF field, the IPG shall pass EMC criteria during and following exposure	ISO/TS 10974 MR imaging environment exposure durations, levels MR imaging EMC acceptance criterion
B0-induced device malfunction limit	14	When exposed to static field, the IPG shall pass EMC criteria during and following exposure	ISO/TS 10974 MR imaging environment exposure durations, levels MR imaging EMC acceptance criterion
Gradient-induced device malfunction limit	16	When exposed to gradient field, the IPG shall pass EMC criteria during and following exposure	ISO/TS 10974 MR imaging environment exposure durations, levels MR imaging EMC acceptance criterion
Combined fields, induced device malfunction limit	17	When exposed to combined static, RF and gradient fields, the IPG shall: Pass EMC criteria during and following exposure Retain its complete functionality during and following exposure	ISO/TS 10974 MR imaging environment exposure durations, levels MR imaging EMC acceptance criterion
Combined fields, image artifacts or distortion		Image artifacts caused by the presence of IPG + leads shall be evaluated per ASTM F2119	ASTM F2119[22]

Abbreviations: CEM 43°C, cumulative number of equivalent minutes at 43°C temperature; EMC, electromagnetic compatibility; N, Newton (force unit); Nm, N m (torque unit); µC, micro Coulomb (charge unit).

> **Table 3**
> **Categorization of MR imaging safety assessments, based on whether or not electromagnetic modeling is involved**
>
> | Six MR Imaging Safety Assessments Rely on Benchtop Testing and/or MR Imaging Scanners Without Modeling | Three MR Imaging Safety Assessments Rely Heavily on Modeling (in Addition to Measurement-Based Testing) |
> |---|---|
> | 1. B0-induced force
2. B0-induced torque
3. Gradient field-induced vibration
4. Gradient field-induced device (IPG) heating
5. Device (IPG) malfunction (B0 field and/or RF field and/or gradient field-induced)
6. Combined fields test | 7. RF field-induced heating of the AIMD
8. Unintended stimulation from RF field-induced lead voltage
9. Unintended stimulation from gradient field-induced lead voltage (extrinsic electric potential) |

B0-Induced Torque

Magnetically induced torque, produced by the static magnetic field (B0), has the potential to cause unwanted movement of a device containing magnetic materials (rotating the implant to align it with the B0 field).

Torque is sensitive to B0 and should be measured at a location where the static magnetic field is homogeneous (eg, the isocenter of an MR scanner). This established test method is described in ASTM F2213,[18] is measurement-based, and is typically conducted in a scanner.

Experimental approaches to conducting torque testing vary in complexity and applicability. Some methodologies are only applicable to devices that experience little to no torque, whereas others are appropriate for devices that experience significant torque and must be more rigorously quantified to assess safety.

Most implantable devices, including AIMDs with extended leads, experience measurable torque but have no trouble passing a reasonable acceptance criterion. There is real potential for concern if the device is in a sensitive physiologic location (eg, brain aneurysm clip).

Gradient Field-Induced Vibration

Time-varying gradient magnetic fields from an MR scanner induce eddy currents on the conductive surfaces of an AIMD. These eddy currents produce a time-varying magnetic moment that interacts with the static magnetic field (B0) causing vibration of the conductive surfaces and, subsequently, the device. The primary potential for patient harm, because the vibration of the device is typically very low-amplitude because of the high frequency of oscillation, arises from possible breakage of internal components that lead to malfunction of the device, which could result in

compromised functionality or lack of therapy from the device.

Vibration is sensitive to B0 and gradient dB/dt. This test is described in ISO/TS 10974:2018,[16] is measurement-based, and is conducted in a scanner or using a shaker table.

There are two methods for testing. One method requires the use of an MR scanner and provides higher accuracy with an increase in test burden, whereas the other method uses a shaker table and uses conservative approximations to reduce test burden after initial calibration testing in an MR scanner. Because most conceived failures are caused by fatigue fractures of internal components, the concept of testing is to expose the implant to extended periods of vibration and confirm full device functionality afterward.

Test duration represents the cumulative patient scan time over the lifetime of a typical AIMD. Guidelines in the standard establish, based on prior clinical experience, that conservative total MR imaging scan time exposure ranges from 2.5 hours to 7.5 hours, if looking at the top 0.8% of the population to the top 0.01% of the population, respectively.

For medium- or small-sized IPGs, and non-life-sustaining devices, vibration is not considered a high-risk hazard. Larger devices typically vibrate more, with potentially greater likelihood of device damage.

Gradient Field-Induced Device (Implanted Pulse Generator) Heating

The time-varying gradient dB/dt fields during MR imaging sequences induce eddy currents on conductive AIMD enclosures and other conductive internal surfaces, such as battery components and circuit ground planes, and can result in device heating.

IPG heating is sensitive to average or root-mean square (RMS) gradient field amplitude |dB/dt|, with secondary dependence on the gradient waveform characteristics (shape and frequency). It is greatest when the device is located where the gradient field |dB/dt| RMS is maximum and when the device is oriented so that the gradient field vector is orthogonal to the AIMD surfaces with the largest conductive area. This heating also scales strongly with device radius (larger devices heat more).

This test is described in ISO/TS 10974:2018.[16] It is measurement-based, with preferential use of a laboratory gradient coil, amplifier, and function generator that can simulate clinical gradient field exposure. Alternatively, testing may be conducted using a clinical MR scanner.

Testing may be conducted using one of two tiers for the gradient waveform shape. Tier 1 uses a conservative waveform shape, and tier 2 allows the characterization and use of a clinically relevant waveform. Tier 2 is most useful for AIMDs with larger conductive surfaces.

The standard calls for a test duration that is the maximum allowed scan duration as specified by the AIMD MR Conditional labeling, or 30 minutes. All other testing parameters are determined by the AIMD manufacturer to reflect conservative clinical use conditions for their device.

The key concern is local tissue heating because of radiant heat from the IPG. For most AIMDs with extended leads, this is not considered a high-risk hazard, although some MR Conditional labels have suggested using an ice pack near a subcutaneous device if the patient reports local heating sensations near the device (IPG).

Device (Implanted Pulse Generator) Malfunction (B0 Field and/or Radiofrequency Field and/or Gradient Field-Induced)

Exposure to the scanner's B0 field and/or RF field and/or gradient field could have certain effects on an AIMD, such as but not limited to:

- B0: Device reset, reprogramming, magnetic remanence, battery drain, and permanent damage.
- B1: Failure to deliver the intended therapy, reprogramming, device reset, permanent damage, and tissue stimulation caused by RF rectification.
- Gradient: Failure to deliver intended therapy, memory corruption, or temporary or permanent loss of device programmed settings.

These effects are transient or permanent and might create a safety hazard that impacts the AIMD patient. Malfunction also has different implications per the patient's dependence on the device (eg, whether it is a life-sustaining therapy, such as a pacemaker, or not).

The assessment is sensitive to a function of B0, peak B1, and peak dB/dt.

Three tests (one per MR field) are described in ISO/TS 10974:2018[16] in elaborate details, including specifying a mixture of radiated and benchtop tests.

- For B0: Implants are divided into three classes with various testing complexities. For many AIMDs with IPG + lead, it is sufficient for their class to meet the test requirement with no specific B0 susceptibility orientations required, and for those, monitoring is done in accordance with a combined field test requirement (eg, the test is done in scanner, with all three fields active).
- For B1 and gradient: The field level and induced voltages are found via a combination of computational modeling (see the later section on modeling) and exposure testing. Challenge testing of the device circuitry for malfunction includes benchtop injected voltage tests using sources of waveforms with appropriate shapes and magnitudes that reflect MR-relevant sequences.

The IPG should pass the acceptance criterion established by the device manufacturer based on the intended functionality (ie, confirm expected device functionality) after the implant is exposed to each one of the three fields as described previously.

Combined Fields Test

The combined fields test provides field exposures typically encountered in clinical MR imaging examinations. It establishes an in vitro evaluation of the AIMD functioning under simultaneous exposure to the static, gradient, and RF magnetic field conditions. Unlike the maximal exposures required in the rest of measurement-based tests, this test exposes the AIMD to representative levels and temporal patterns of all three MR magnetic fields simultaneously.

This measurement-based assessment is conducted in a scanner and is sensitive to (a function of) B0, RF peak, and dB/dt Peak. The test is described in ISO/TS 10974:2018.[16]

The combined fields test is performed using an AIMD (the IPG and the connected leads) positioned in a tissue-simulating media phantom and placed inside an MR scanner. The AIMD is exposed to a series of MR imaging sequences (representing various common and clinically relevant protocols) performed at different landmarks or simulated patient positions within the bore. The concept of testing is to expose the implant to the clinical combined fields and confirm expected device functionality during and after the exposure.

This test is viewed as redundant to device (IPG) malfunction testing. However, it is required to make sure the device is actually tested in radiated environment under clinical conditions. In addition, benchtop exposure tests are typically more stringent, because they can apply higher-than-expected injection levels.

MR IMAGING SAFETY ASSESSMENTS WITH ELECTROMAGNETIC MODELING

ISO/TS 10974:2018[16] has tiered approaches to modeling where the low tier is easily implementable but overestimates the needed assessment, and modeling in higher tiers is more complex but more accurate (with less overestimation). Practically, for AIMDs with extended leads, tier 3 is the highest tier that is attainable with acceptable accuracy.

Tier 3 includes modeling the EM environment surrounding the AIMD to obtain the incident electric fields potentially picked up by the AIMD, together with measurements of how the AIMD handles such incident fields.

The process includes running a computer simulation: using a hardware model of the scanner coil itself, whether an RF birdcage coil or a gradient coil, and anatomic models of humans as representative samples per the device's patient characteristics. EM simulations (RF or gradient) are run using these models in all relevant clinical landmarks or patient positions to mimic the EM environment of the scanner. Modern simulations, across a range of human body models, and with a range of MR imaging scanner coil models, can give the EM field distribution everywhere inside the anatomic models across a range of potential MR examination circumstances.

The First Element Needed for Modeling, Tangential Electric Fields

For the three assessments that rely heavily on modeling (see **Table 3**), tier 3 modeling requires that, along the lead path in every anatomic model, the tangential vector of the electrical component (E-tan) of the incident fields be extracted from the EM simulation. **Fig. 3** shows the E-tan magnitude of example DBS and Spinal Cord Stimulation (SCS) routings, for a specific landmark in an MR scanner with an RF body coil.

The Second Element Needed for Modeling, the Transfer Function

For RF (the first two of the three assessments in **Table 3**) the transfer function[19] is needed, which is really a characterization of how a particular AIMD (ie, a specific IPG + lead combination) behaves as an RF Antenna in the scanner environment.

For safety purposes benefiting the patient, we want the AIMD to be a bad antenna in the EM environment of the MR imaging scanner. The transfer function of an AIMD (when exposed to a uniform E-tan excitation) is measured in benchtop RF injected setup (**Fig. 4**) or simulated. The transfer function is a 1D vector (having the length of the lead under test) of complex values (term S in Equations 1 and 2) whose magnitude shows the resonance lengths of the AIMD (see **Fig. 5**), which is the frequencies at which the AIMD is a good antenna.

Discussed next are the three MR safety assessments that rely on modeling.

Radiofrequency Field-Induced Heating of the Active Implantable Medical Device (Lead Electrode Heating)

Patient harm caused by RF-induced lead electrode heating is a function of absolute temperature, duration of the temperature, and individual

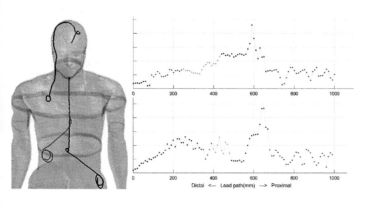

Fig. 3. (*Left*) Human model with two DBS and two SCS lead routings (pathways). (*Upper Right*) RF E-tan magnitude of one DBS routing. (*Lower Right*) RF E-tan magnitude of one SCS routing.

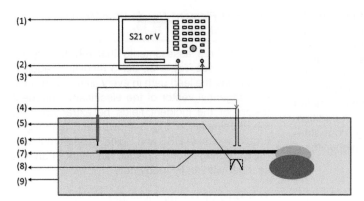

Fig. 4. The transfer function bench-top RF injected setup: Vector Network Analyzer (1), RF source (2), sense input (3), transmitting antenna (4), localized E-tan (z) (5), coaxial antenna (6), tip electrode (7), the AIMD (lead + IPG) (8), and tissue simulating phantom (9). (*From* ISO TIR 21900:2018. Guidance for uncertainty analysis regarding the application of ISO/TS 10974; with permission.)

implant considerations. The assessment is sensitive to (a function of) B1 RMS, and the test method is described in ISO/TS 10974:2018.[16]

The concept of this assessment is:

- Benchtop/scanner: The AIMD (the IPG and the connected leads) is positioned in a tissue-simulating media phantom and placed inside an RF birdcage (designed for testing or of a scanner) and lead electrode heating is measured under various incident field conditions (multiple lead pathways and/or RF exposures).
- Simulation: Using simulation of this benchtop setup (in vitro), the E-tans are extracted for all clinical lead pathways.
- Benchtop or simulation: The transfer function of the AIMD is measured in benchtop injected setup or simulated.
- A predictive model of heating (and/or power) is established using the dot product of

E-tans and transfer function per the following formula[19]:

$$P = A \left| \int_0^l S_{hotspot}(z) E_{tan}(z) dz \right|^2 \qquad \textbf{Equation 1}$$

Where P is power (or heating), A is scaler imbedding the linear fit of the AIMD model and the incident field levels, S is the transfer function, E-tans are the in vitro tangential electrical incident fields, and dz is the spatial distance increment along lead length.

- The previous formula, which describes how the AIMD model is derived, is also applied to the extracted E-tans of the human (in vivo) simulations. This often results in thousands to millions of heating predictions, accounting

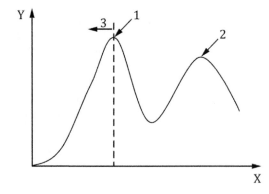

Fig. 5. When the AIMD is exposed to a uniform E-tan excitation, the transfer function is obtained via measurements in benchtop RF injected setup or simulation. The peaks in its magnitude represent resonance lengths. The example here shows two resonance lengths. (*From* ISO/TS 10974:2018. Assessment of the safety of magnetic resonance imaging for patients with an active implantable medical device; with permission.)

Key

1   first resonance
2   second resonance
3   below resonance
X   AIMD length
Y   deposited power at hotspot

for all clinical lead pathway scenarios and imaging conditions (human models, RF coils, and landmarks).

- Experimental exposure tests yield normalization factors that tie the heating results to specific B1 + RMS levels, allowing prediction of heating under any desired B1 + RMS, and MR imaging normal mode or first level mode Specific Absorption Rate (SAR) conditions.
- The heating acceptance criterion for the tissue surrounding the electrodes dictates what RF limit is appropriate for this specific AIMD.
  - If the results of this assessment determine that this particular AIMD lead electrodes heat up tissue surrounding the electrodes up to X degrees Celsius under MR imaging normal mode SAR, and if the acceptance criterion threshold for these tissues heating is greater than this X level, then scanning under normal mode is safe for this AIMD.
  - However, if the acceptance criterion for these tissues heating is lower than this X level, then safe scanning requires dialing down the RF level in the scanner environment to lower than the MR imaging normal mode limit, all the way to the level at which heating is lower than the acceptance criterion threshold. That RF exposure level will be deemed acceptable and will be expressed in B1 + RMS (and its corresponding SAR) as the RF limit in the MR Conditional list of the device label.

Unintended Stimulation from Radiofrequency Field-Induced Rectified Lead Voltage

This assessment is similar to the lead electrode heating. However, it is sensitive to (a function of) B1 peak. The test is described in ISO/TS 10974:2018.[16]

The concept of this assessment is as follows:

- Benchtop/scanner: The AIMD (the IPG and the connected leads) is positioned in a tissue-simulating media phantom and placed inside an RF birdcage (designed for testing or of a scanner) and lead injection voltage toward the IPG is measured under various incident field conditions (multiple lead pathways and/or RF exposures).
- Simulation: Using simulation of this benchtop setup (in vitro), the E-tans are extracted for all clinical lead pathways.
- Benchtop or simulation: The transfer function of the AIMD is measured in benchtop injected setup or simulated.
- A predictive model of injection voltage is established using the dot product of E-tans

and transfer function per the following formula:

$$V = A \int_0^l S(z) E_{tan}(z) dz \qquad \textbf{Equation 2}$$

Where V is the voltage level, A is scaler imbedding the linear fit of the AIMD model and the incident field levels, S is the transfer function, E-tans are the in vitro tangential electrical incident fields, and dz is the spatial distance increment along lead length.

- The previous formula, which describes how the AIMD model is derived, is also applied to the extracted E-tans of the human (in vivo) simulations. That results in thousands to millions of RF level predictions accounting for all clinical lead pathway scenarios and imaging conditions (human models, RF coils, and landmarks).
- The proper B1 peak values reflecting various RF coil types in clinical scanners are used in this assessment.
- The IPG should pass the acceptance criterion established by the device manufacturer based on the intended functionality when this voltage level is injected into the IPG.

Unintended Stimulation from Gradient Field-Induced Lead Voltage (Extrinsic Electric Potential)

Various scenarios of intralead, interlead, or between electrodes and a conductive IPG enclosure can result in current flow through the IPG and could cause unintended stimulation to tissue in contact with the electrodes. This assessment is similar to the RF field-induced rectified lead voltage. However, per the nature of gradient fields, it does not rely on a transfer function. The assessment is sensitive to (a function of) dB/dt peak. The test is described in ISO/TS 10974:2018.[16]

The concept of this assessment is as follows:

- The injection voltage assessment is established using the extracted E-tans of the human (in vivo) gradient simulations:

$$V = \int E \cdot dl \qquad \textbf{Equation 3}$$

Where V is the voltage level, E are the in vitro tangential electrical incident fields, and dl is the spatial distance increment along lead length.

- That results in thousands to millions of voltage predictions accounting for all clinical lead pathway scenarios and imaging conditions (human models, gradient coils, and landmarks).
- The IPG should pass the acceptance criterion established by the device manufacturer based on the intended functionality when this voltage is injected into the IPG.

Learning points for radiologists on scanning patients safely per implant MR labels:

- For an MR Conditional AIMD, the labeling conditions take care of the safety issues as long as clinical conditions stay within them per the device MR imaging instructions for use. That is, the clinical team does not need to deal with specific AIMD-MR risk-benefit decisions, if the conditions are be met as per the MR Conditional labels.
- Some implants allow scanning under the MR imaging scanner normal mode, which does not usually pose a challenge to MR technologists in performing safe and effective examinations.
- Other implants may have limits on time-varying gradients (not likely) and/or RF, which is the most common limit (typically expressed as B1 + RMS and/or SAR limits).
- Implants with a zonal (landmark) restriction typically have a restriction based on sensitivity to B1 + RMS.
- Implants with coil-type restriction (eg, a head coil–only MR label) are also related to RF restriction based on sensitivity to B1 + RMS (although B1 peak is different for various coils). Head-only Tx coils expose the patients to RF fields only within the head coil. In devices only cleared for head coil transmission, if the RF body coil activates, or if the RF coil is a receive-only head coil, it could present a significant patient hazard.
- For those implants with RF limit of B1 + RMS (and its corresponding SAR limit), using the B1 + RMS based limit is better (less restrictive), provided the scanner shows B1 + RMS. This is because the SAR limit is the minimum value for the range of SAR values corresponding to this one B1 + RMS limit (ie, for each B1 + RMS value, the corresponding SAR is a range because SAR is a function of body weight and landmark).
- Not obeying the RF limits of MR Conditional label can lead to exceeding the acceptable limit for patient harms that are sensitive to B1 + RMS/SAR and/or RF coil type

restrictions and/or zone landmark restrictions, most importantly electrode heating. The most prominent example, documented in 2005, is a DBS patient who was scanned in violation of multiple labeling conditions, leading to a permanent neurologic deficit.[8]

- Device malfunctions are related to B0 field strength, or B1 peak or dB/dt peak levels, parameters that cannot readily be altered presently by an MR technologist in the clinic. Thus, it is important to abide by the MR imaging conditions defined in the label for safe scanning.
- For AIMDs requiring setting up the device in MR imaging mode before scanning, it is important to do so to avoid potential device malfunctions that can occur either during or following MR imaging exposure.
- For AIMDs requiring RF lower than normal mode when the pulse sequence to be used exceeds the implant B1 + RMS/SAR limit,
  ○ If the scanner is implant friendly, use the recommended option/software. A good example of that is Philips Healthcare (Amsterdam, the Netherlands) ScanWise Implant system.[20] Otherwise, any parameter that affects RF can be adjusted to reduce RF.
  ○ Use the "Low SAR" option. It is available on most scanners and helps to reduce B1 + RMS/SAR, typically without impacting image quality significantly. Always use this option in combination with one or more options from the following:
  ○ Increase TR (not to the extent of changing contrast, as in T1-SE sequences), and/or,
  ○ Reduce the number of slices (slice grouping), and/or,
  ○ Reduce flip-angle (alpha), reduce refocusing flip angle, or using fewer RF saturation bands.
  ○ Reduce the number of echoes (echo train length/turbo factor/shot factor).

SUMMARY

MR Conditional labels for AIMDs are developed through rigorous testing by implantable device manufacturers, using methods and guidelines that were developed with contributions from experts in various fields including MR scanner manufacturers, implant manufacturers, and regulatory agencies. Formal instructions for use of MR Conditional implants are the proper source for MR scanning conditions and parameters that can ensure patient safety. The MR imaging safety community is gaining expertise from the use of more MR

Conditional AIMDs and reflecting these learnings with collaborations from experts in the field for the benefit and safety of scanning patients with implants. Patients and clinicians have also benefitted from efforts by MR manufacturers to design more advanced MR imaging scanners and software, including those with options for limiting exposure fields. These have already helped clinicians to provide access to MR imaging for patients with implanted devices, and there are exciting opportunities for improving patient safe access in the future through advancing technologies and continued collaboration in the development of safety testing methods and standards.

REFERENCES

1. IEC 60601-2-33:2010+AMD1:2013+AMD2:2015 CSV, Consolidated version. Medical electrical equipment - Part 2-33: Particular requirements for the basic safety and essential performance of magnetic resonance equipment for medical diagnosis.
2. Delfino JG, Krainak DM, Flesher SA, et al. MRI-related FDA adverse event reports: a 10-yr review. Med Phys 2019;46(12):5562–71.
3. Erlebacher JA, Cahill PT, Pannizzo F, et al. Effect of magnetic resonance imaging on DDD pacemakers. Am J Cardiol 1986;57(6):437–40.
4. Becker RL, Norfray JF, Teitelbaum GP, et al. MR imaging in patients with intracranial aneurysm clips. AJNR Am J Neuroradiol 1988;9(5):885–9.
5. Klucznik RP, Carrier DA, Pyka R, et al. Placement of a ferromagnetic intracerebral aneurysm clip in a magnetic field with a fatal outcome. Radiology 1993;187(3):855–6.
6. Fagan LL, Shellock FG, Brenner RJ, et al. Ex vivo evaluation of ferromagnetism, heating, and artifacts of breast tissue expanders exposed to a 1.5-T MR system. J Magn Reson Imaging 1995;5(5):614–6.
7. Hess T, Stepanow B, Knopp MV. Safety of intrauterine contraceptive devices during MR imaging. Eur Radiol 1996;6(1):66–8.
8. Henderson JM, Tkach J, Phillips M, et al. Permanent neurological deficit related to magnetic resonance imaging in a patient with implanted deep brain stimulation electrodes for Parkinson's disease: case report. Neurosurgery 2005;57(5):E1063.
9. ASTM F2182 - 19e2. Standard test method for measurement of radio frequency induced heating on or near passive implants during magnetic resonance imaging.
10. ASTM F2503-20. Standard practice for marking medical devices and other items for safety in the magnetic resonance environment.
11. Shellock FG, Kanal E. Magnetic resonance: bioeffects, safety, and patient management. New York: Raven Press; 1994.
12. Shellock FG. Pocket guide to MR procedures and metallic objects: update 1994. New York: Raven Press; 1994.
13. ISO 14708-1:2014. Implants for surgery — Active implantable medical devices — Part 1: General requirements for safety, marking and for information to be provided by the manufacturer.
14. Mitka M. First MRI-safe pacemaker receives conditional approval from FDA. JAMA 2011;305(10): 985–6.
15. ISO/TS 10974:2012. Assessment of the safety of magnetic resonance imaging for patients with an active implantable medical device.
16. ISO/TS 10974:2018. Assessment of the safety of magnetic resonance imaging for patients with an active implantable medical device.
17. ASTM F2052-15. Standard test method for measurement of magnetically induced displacement force on medical devices in the magnetic resonance environment.
18. ASTM F2213-17. Standard test method for measurement of magnetically induced torque on medical devices in the magnetic resonance environment.
19. Park SM, Kamondetdacha R, Nyenhuis JA. Calculation of MRI-induced heating of an implanted medical lead wire with an electric field transfer function. J Magn Reson Imaging 2007;26(5):1278–85.
20. Available at: https://www.usa.philips.com/healthcare/education-resources/technologies/mri/scanwise-implant. Accessed July 18, 2020.
21. Kainz W. MR heating tests of MR critical implants. J Magn Reson Imaging 2007;26(3):450–1.
22. ASTM F2119 - 07(2013). Standard test method for evaluation of MR image artifacts from passive implants.

Magnetic Resonance Safety in the 7T Environment

Andrew J. Fagan, PhD*, Kimberly K. Amrami, MD, Kirk M. Welker, MD,
Matthew A. Frick, MD, Joel P. Felmlee, PhD, Robert E. Watson Jr, MD, PhD

KEYWORDS

- 7T MR imaging • Bioeffects • Vestibular activation • Parallel transmit • Image artifacts
- Local specific absorption rate • Simulations

KEY POINTS

- The higher static field gives rise to slightly increased translational and torque forces on paramagnetic and ferromagnetic objects.
- Bioeffects are also increased, in particular vestibular activation which can produce transitory dizziness and vertigo in patients entering and exiting the scanner.
- MR conditional implants at 3T may be unsafe to scan at 7T, due to potential for unsafe magnetic forces and RF-induced heating.
- Institutional safety policies and procedures should be developed and maintained to adhere to best practice by a dedicated 7T Safety Team.
- Staff training is required to address challenges specific to operating in a 7T environment and to interpret the altered image contrast and artifact appearance.

INTRODUCTION

Ensuring safety in the 7T MR imaging environment shares many of the considerations that pertain to lower magnetic field strength MR imaging systems, although interactions with the higher static magnetic fields and higher frequency electromagnetic energy pose additional challenges. These interactions with the body give rise predominately to enhanced bioeffects, a potential for specific absorption rate (SAR) hotspots, and image quality problems.[1,2] Similarly, interactions with conductive and/or magnetic objects in Zone 4, implanted or otherwise, increase the risk of injury caused by magnetic forces acting on these objects, and may also increase the potential for SAR hotspots via induced electric fields adjacent to conductive implants. Understanding the origins of such effects is key to developing strategies to minimize the risk they pose and thereby ensure safety of patients and research subjects.

7T MR imaging technology has undergone continual development over the past approximately 20 years since the first magnet was installed.[3] In 2003, the US Food and Drug Administration (FDA) declared that MR imaging up to 8T constitutes a nonsignificant risk for adults, children, and infants 1 month of age and older. The 2015 amendment of the International Electrotechnical Commission (IEC) 60601-2-33 standard subsequently increased the first-level controlled operating mode for the static magnetic field to 8T.[4] In 2017, a first system achieved regulatory clearance in Europe and the United States for patient diagnostic imaging, albeit for brain and

Department of Radiology, Mayo Clinic, 200 First Street Southwest, Rochester, MN 55905, USA
* Corresponding author.
E-mail address: Fagan.Andrew@mayo.edu

Magn Reson Imaging Clin N Am 28 (2020) 573–582
https://doi.org/10.1016/j.mric.2020.07.002
1064-9689/20/© 2020 Elsevier Inc. All rights reserved.

extremity imaging only. At the time of writing, there are over 80 7T MR imaging systems installed around the world, and although most these are located in research facilities, the number of systems operating in clinical environments is growing rapidly.

This article will outline the safety considerations specific to the 7T MR imaging clinical environment. Safety aspects of new 7T technologies currently under development in research laboratories and which can be expected to impact clinical 7T MR imaging in the coming years will also be discussed.

FORCES CAUSED BY STATIC MAGNETIC FIELDS AND MAGNETIC FIELD GRADIENTS
Spatial Field Gradients

The current regulatory cleared clinical 7T MR imaging system has an actively shielded magnet

and a consequent footprint that is only slightly larger than conventional lower-field systems. Magnetic field contour lines are plotted in **Fig. 1**, comparing the fringe fields of this system to that of a conventional actively-shielded 3T system. The 7T contour lines extend further from the magnet, and the spatial field gradients (SFGs) are similar if not slightly lower in this fringe field area. Inside the bore, the situation is similar: the maximum SFG in a patient-accessible area in this 7T magnet is 12.2 T/m, compared with the maximum values reported on conventional actively shielded cylindrical horizontal-bore 1.5T and 3T magnets (19.0 and 17.0 T/m, respectively[5]). As a result, the Lenz force acting on electrically conductive implants moving through the magnet's SFGs is lower on this 7T system, since this force only depends on the magnitude of the spatial field gradients for a given velocity of movement through the SFG. Older 7T MR imaging

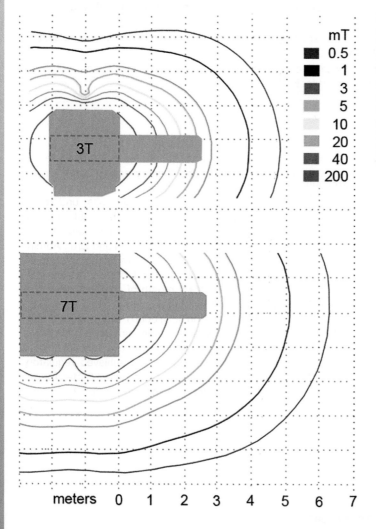

Fig. 1. Schematic showing the magnetic field contour lines in the fringe field region in front of the current regulatory-cleared 7T system (Magnetom Terra, Siemens Medical Systems, Germany), compared with that of a conventional 3T system (Prisma, Siemens Medical Systems). The slightly wider-spacing of the field lines for the 7T system indicate a lower spatial field gradient in this fringe field region.

mT
0.5
1
3
5
10
20
40
200

3T

7T

meters 0 1 2 3 4 5 6 7

systems, and indeed future 7T magnet designs, may of course differ in this regard, but nevertheless SFGs are of less concern for current 7T technology.

Translational Forces

The translational force exerted on an unsaturated para- or ferromagnetic object is directly related to the product of the static field and the SFG at that point. In general, the static field strength at the spatial location where the maximum SFG occurs depends on the magnet design. For the regulatory cleared 7T magnet, the maximum SFG of 12.2 T/m occurs near the inner bore wall, approximately 1 m from isocenter (but still 0.5 m in from the bore opening) where the static field is approximately 5 T. This results in a maximum [static field x SFG] product of 61.1 T^2/m. The maximum values for lower field cylindrical horizontal bore magnets are typically less than 50 T^2/m, and hence these magnets will exert a correspondingly lower translational force on unsaturated para- or ferromagnetic objects. It is worth noting, however, that some high-field open (HFO) magnet designs exceed the [static field x SFG] product of current 7T magnets in patient-accessible areas, and hence will exert stronger translational forces on objects at those specific locations.

Force due to Torque

The force due to torque exerted on unsaturated para- or ferromagnetic objects scales linearly with the strength of the static magnetic field, and hence it will exceed that on a 3T magnet by a factor of approximately 2.3. Thin, elongated objects such as long orthopedic rods may be of particular concern in this regard.[6]

Metallic Implants

The potential for unsafe forces of translation and torque on metallic implants in patients must be carefully evaluated before imaging at 7T. At the time of writing, only a handful of implants have been certified as magnetic resonance conditional at 7T by the device manufacturers, principally small middle ear and intraocular implants made of titanium.[7–10] All other implants have no such certification at present, and it is unclear whether manufacturers will expend the necessary resources in the near future to certify their implants given the relatively small installed base of 7T systems and difficulty in accessing 7T systems for testing. The imaging of patients with most metallic implants is therefore performed off-label, and as such requires careful evaluation of the risk/benefit

to the patient. There are several studies in the peer-reviewed scientific literature describing magnetic forces on a range of metallic implants. These include studies of dental retainer wires and implants,[11,12] orthopedic devices,[13,14] cranial fixation devices,[15] middle ear implants,[16] intrauterine devices,[14,17] cardiac and vascular stents,[13,18] and intracranial aneurysm clips.[19] For most of the devices investigated, no significant magnetic forces were reported, although 2 stents,[13] 1 long orthopedic implant,[13] a dental magnetic attachment keeper,[12] and 1 intracranial aneurysm and 1 hemostatic clip[19] did exhibit potentially dangerous effects. Furthermore, 2 shunt valves could not be programmed after exposure to a 7T field.[20]

For implants for which no unsafe forces were reported, these data can be used to inform risk/benefit analyses conducted on individual patients for whom 7T MR imaging has been prescribed and who have these specific devices implanted. Care should be exercised when extrapolating data on specific devices to other devices even if nominally similar, given the critical dependence of the device's material composition on the magnitude of any forces.[13]

Effects caused by switching imaging magnetic field gradients

The switching of imaging magnetic field gradients on current-generation 7T MR imaging systems has similar performance characteristics (typically, amplitude of 80 mT/m and slew rate of 200 T/m/s) as conventional high-end 3T systems, and hence incidences of peripheral nerve stimulation are no greater at 7T. One might expect the acoustic noise to be greater at 7T because of the increased Lorentz force exerted on the gradient coils. However, the experience is of broadly similar acoustic noise levels, The 2 highest acoustic noise levels on the authors' 7T system (Magnetom Terra) were measured for fMR imaging and B_0 mapping sequences (LAeq = 102.4 and 103.4 dBA, respectively). This may be due to several factors, such as an increased Lorentz damping effect,[21] additional acoustic insulation in the magnet bore (where a body coil would typically be located), and perhaps also a greater damping mass of the magnet itself. However, the only current regulatory cleared 7T head coil (1Tx/32Rx, Nova Medical Inc.) has a narrower inner diameter compared with most head coils on lower field systems, making it impractical to use headphones for additional acoustic protection.

Vibrations within highly conductive implants caused by eddy current-induced torque are likely to be greater at 7T than at lower fields. Although these could potentially produce uncomfortable sensations in patients (eg, with cardiac stents), it is unclear whether this is the case and whether these would pose a safety concern.

Other Bioeffects

There is no evidence in the scientific literature describing any long-term bioeffect on people because of exposure to 7T static magnetic fields, reflecting the 2015 amendment to the 60601-2-33 standard allowing for fields up to 8T.[4,22] However, short-term, transient effects are elevated at 7T compared with lower fields. For example, the Lorentz force acting on the positively and negatively charged ions in the blood is greater at 7T. This magnetohydrodynamic effect generates an electric field that alters the pattern of electrocardiograms (ECGs), predominately manifest as an elevated T-wave. No other significant effects on the cardiovascular system (eg, changes to heart rate, blood pressure, or cardiac output) have been reported at 7T.

Other induced voltages give rise to activation of the vestibular apparatus in the inner ear, resulting in feelings of dizziness, vertigo, and moving on a curve, particularly on entering and leaving the magnet.[23–25] Several mechanisms have been proposed as the source of this phenomenon, predominate of which is the Lorentz force generated by the interaction between normal ionic currents in the inner ear endolymph and the large static and gradient magnetic fields.[26] Thus, although exposure to the 7T field while stationary at the isocenter can cause such vestibular activations, the most severe effect is generally reported by patients and research subjects to occur when moving into the magnet, although the experience is highly subjective (30%–85% of individuals report such activations to varying degrees).[1,23] In the vast majority of cases, feelings of dizziness or postural instability return to baseline within several minutes of exiting the magnet.[24] In rare cases, the vestibular activation can lead to nausea, although this appears to be strongly correlated with moving through areas of particularly high spatial field gradients (perhaps greater than approximately 10 T/m) within the magnet bore, which on the current regulatory-cleared 7T scanner only occurs when the patient's head is positioned more than approximately 15 to 20 cm away from the magnet axis (side-to-side, or lifted off the table). Incidences of further bioeffects such as metallic taste and

magnetophosphenes are similar to those reported at lower fields.

EFFECTS CAUSED BY HIGH RESONANT FREQUENCIES AT 7T
Interaction of 300 MHz RF Energy with Tissue

The resonant (Larmor) frequency for ^{1}H nuclei at 7T is 300 MHz, which poses several safety challenges for imaging at 7T. The interaction of 300 MHz energy with the body is more complex than at lower frequencies, because the wavelengths of these radiofrequency photons are similar or less than typical body dimensions. These wavelengths vary considerably from tissue to tissue, depending on the dielectric properties (permittivity and conductivity) of the tissue itself, and range from 10 cm in fluids to 40 cm in fat. As a consequence, it is difficult to produce a uniform RF transmit field within the body, because of complex patterns of constructive and destructive interference created within the tissue, which can vary widely even across structures as small as the head or knee. This can potentially result in SAR hotspots. It furthermore results in nonuniform flip angles across the field of view, which can negatively impact image contrast. This is particularly problematic for large, body-sized birdcage coil designs, which are consequently not used on 7T systems. Rather, the regulatory cleared 7T imaging of the brain and knee is performed using dedicated transmit/receive coils, whose birdcage transmit coils are at the upper limit of useful size at 300 MHz. To image larger body areas at 7T, such as the pelvis, abdomen, and torso, new transmit coil design concepts are required, typically based on arrays of individual loops or dipole antennae that can each be driven by a separate RF amplifier (in parallel transmit mode).[27–29] Indeed, the imaging of smaller fields of view will also benefit enormously from parallel transmit technology in terms of SAR reduction and image quality improvements. However, at the time of writing, parallel transmit technology has not achieved regulatory clearance for diagnostic imaging,[1,30] although significant effort is being expended to address this challenge.

Local Specific Absorption Rate Supervision

RF-induced tissue heating is a concern when imaging at all field strengths, and is typically controlled via limits on the SAR during the imaging session. At 3T and lower, global SAR limits are used to constrain the RF power deposition in tissue. Global SAR values are averaged over the whole or partial body (such as the head). At 7T, 10 g local SAR limits must also be enforced; these

Table 1
Global and local specific absorption rate limits, adapted from the IEC[4]

	Normal	1st Level Controlled	2nd Level Controlled
Global SAR [W/kg]			
Whole body	2	4	>4
Partial body	2–10	4–10	>4–10
Head	3.2	3.2	>3.2
Local SAR [W/kg]			
Trunk	10	20	>20
Limbs	20	40	>40

The limits are listed for an averaging time of 6 min. Global SAR limits apply to volume transmit coils, while the local SAR limits apply for local transmit coils.
Adapted from Fiedler TM, Ladd ME, Bitz AK. SAR Simulations & Safety. *Neuroimage.* 2018;168:33-58 with permission.

are presented in **Table 1**. In general, limits on local SAR are more restrictive than global SAR, which can be understood qualitatively by reference to the electromagnetic simulation in **Fig. 2**. This simulation shows the 10 g local SAR distribution in a virtual head produced by RF energy transmitted from a standard circularly polarized birdcage coil at 64, 128, and 300 MHz. At all frequencies, it is apparent that an SAR hotspot exists toward the top of the head for this transmit coil configuration. The 10 W/kg SAR_{10g} limit (20 W/kg in first-level controlled mode) is consistently

reached at this location much sooner than the 3.2 W/kg SAR_{global} limit. A further compounding factor for imaging at 7T, particularly for RF-intense sequences such as turbo spin echo, derives from the quadratic dependence of SAR on B_0 (ie, SAR $\propto B_0^2$), and hence a factor 5.4 times more RF energy is required to achieve a given flip angle at 7T compared with 3T.

A consequence of the supervision of local SAR at 7T is the need to use electromagnetic simulations to estimate the RF heating induced in the body. The global SAR for a particular imaging

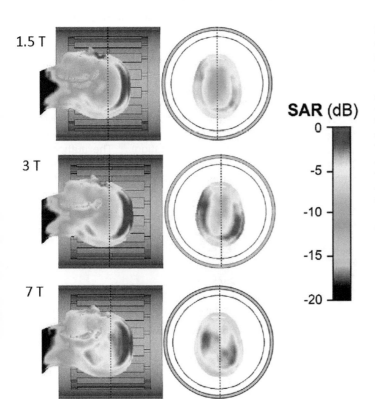

1.5 T

3 T

7 T

SAR (dB)

0

-5

-10

-15

-20

Fig. 2. Electromagnetic simulations comparing the local SAR distribution produced in the head at 1.5T, 3T, and 7T (corresponding to 64 MHz, 128 MHz, and 300 MHz, respectively). At all field strengths, a SAR hotspot exists toward the top of the head, with a more complex pattern emerging as the frequency increases. The head-averaged SAR levels at 3T and lower minimize the impact of these hotspots. At 7T, where limits on local 10 g local SAR are enforced, these hotspots play an increasingly important role. (*Adapted from* Fiedler TM, Ladd ME, Bitz AK. SAR Simulations & Safety. Neuroimage 2018;168:33-58 with permission.)

sequence can be determined directly from real-time measurement of the overall magnitude of RF power reflected from the body transmit coil during RF transmission. However, such RF power measurements cannot provide any information on the spatial distribution of SAR within the body, which is necessary for local SAR determination. The numerical simulations must be capable of solving Maxwell's equations at every point within a virtual representation of the human body, and several virtual phantoms exist for this purpose.[31] These calculations take many hours to compute, even with computer workstations equipped with the best graphical processing units, because of their complexity and the need to perform the calculations at every point within the virtual phantom and extending out beyond a virtual representation of the RF coil itself. As such, they are impracticable to run for each patient, but rather worse case scenarios are precalculated in simulations for the particular RF coil configuration. These scenarios are then used to constrain the RF power that can be transmitted into the body for all patients, resulting in a necessarily conservative RF transmit power used for most patients. Several methods are under development to accelerate the calculation of the B_1^+ and electric fields, and hence SAR distributions, generated by the RF coil by reducing the number of calculations that need to be performed via compression algorithms such as virtual observation points.[32,33] These methods hold potential for tailoring the RF transmit power to each patient, although further evaluation of safety is required to ensure local SAR levels remain within regulatory limits.

Conductive Implants

Any conductive material, whether implanted in the body or on the skin surface (eg, tattoos or jewelry), will further alter the local SAR distribution, and hence the scanning of patients with such materials requires particular attention at 7T. A limited number of publications have investigated RF-induced heating of various implants at 7T, including dental implants,[11] orthopedic fixation devices,[13] cranial fixation plates and devices,[15,34,35] stents,[18,36,37] aneurysm clips,[19,38,39] intrauterine devices,[17,40] and electroencephalogram leads.[41] Some studies used phantom-based experiments to measure temperature increases using fiber-optic sensors, but more recent approaches favor simulation-based approaches. Simulations can better replicate the heterogeneity within the body, and also deal with different configurations (eg, body habitus, implant positioning relative to tissue structures and coil, or different transmit coil modes). **Fig. 3** compares the vastly different SAR distributions that are generated in homogeneous and heterogeneous objects, illustrating the need to perform simulations using models that adequately replicate anatomy. Such simulations can also provide information on both SAR and tissue temperature (this latter via thermal simulations using models of blood perfusion).[11,36,38] In the studies reported to date, SAR levels were found to increase, sometimes several-fold, close to the implants, but in general remained below regulatory levels for the specific experimental/simulation set-ups investigated. Data from one representative experiment are presented in **Fig. 4**. In one study of cranial fixation plates, the SAR hotspot occurred distant from the implant and hence was not impacted by the presence of the device.[34] In a further study, the orientation of a stent relative to the local electric field (whose direction is extremely difficult to predict in the body) was also found to impact the local SAR, with unsafe increases measured in certain conditions (eg, aneurysm clip length and orientation).[38] The authors also reported simulated values of 1 g local SAR and tissue temperature, since SAR values averaged

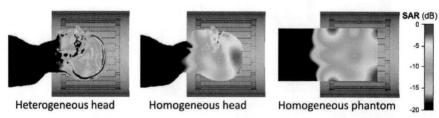

Heterogeneous head   Homogeneous head   Homogeneous phantom

Fig. 3. Electromagnetic simulations showing the voxel-wise SAR distributions generated in 3 objects: a heterogeneous head model containing different tissue types, a homogeneous head model containing a uniform tissue-equivalent material, and a cylindrical homogeneous phantom also containing a uniform tissue-equivalent material The significant differences in SAR patterns illustrate the need to perform simulations using models that adequately replicate anatomy. (*Adapted from* Fiedler TM, Ladd ME, Bitz AK. SAR Simulations & Safety. *Neuroimage.* 2018;168:33-58 with permission.)

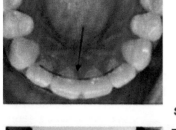

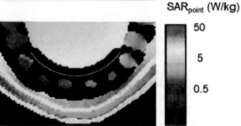

SAR$_{point}$ (W/kg)

50

5

0.5

Fig. 4. Example of experiments aimed at assessing RF-induced heating due to the presence of permanent dental retainer wires at 7T. Physical experiments performed in uniform phantoms using fiber optic temperature measurements were supplemented with detailed electromagnetic simulations of the SAR distribution. (*Adapted from* Wezel J, Kooij BJ, Webb AG. Assessing the MR compatibility of dental retainer wires at 7 Tesla. Magn Reson Med. 2014;72(4):1191-1198 with permission.)

over a relatively large 10 g of tissue may not adequately ensure safety for implants with narrow geometric features, where focal SAR hotspots may occur.

The data presented in such studies can be used to inform risk/benefit analyses for individual patients in similar circumstances (ie, with respect to implanted device type, position within the body, and RF transmit coil). Nevertheless, care should be exercised in extrapolating to dissimilar conditions. The potential for RF heating because of conductive materials decreases significantly when the materials are located away from the RF transmit field.[14] The lack of a body coil on the current regulatory cleared 7T system, and hence more localized nature of the RF transmit field from the head and knee coils, can thus be used to inform the risk/benefit analysis. A caveat here is the traveling wave phenomena, which, at 300 MHz, can result in some RF energy propagating along the bore of the magnet and hence delivering RF energy to body areas distant from the coil.[42] At their institution, the authors have scanned over 200 patients/subjects with implanted devices located both within and outside the RF transmit field, including: cranial fixation plates, orthodontic devices (braces, bridges, crowns, pivot teeth, retainers), orthopedic devices (hip/knee replacements, spinal fusion/compression plates, rods, screws, nails),

intrauterine devices, surgical clips, vascular prostheses, and ports.

The previous discussion relates to passive devices; at present, there are no data in the literature on imaging of subjects with active implants at 7T.

High-Permittivity Dielectric Pads

A commonly used method to improve uniformity in 7T images is through the use of high electric permittivity dielectric pads, typically manufactured from perovskite ceramic powders mixed with D_2O to for a thick slurry.[43,44] These pads create a local focusing of the transmitted B_1 field close to the pads, resulting in a more uniform flip angle distribution across the field of view.[45,46] The presence of such pads is not typically included in the algorithms used to supervise local SAR, and hence several studies have investigated their effect on SAR distributions in such situations. Data suggest a minor effect on SAR, in many cases effecting a reduction in the RF power required to achieve the desired B_1 field strength in the region of interest, and hence a lowering SAR over the entire exposed region.[44] The use of dielectric pads should nevertheless be used with reference to studies describing their effects when used in similar conditions.

PRACTICAL CONSIDERATIONS
Magnetic Resonance Safety Team

Ensuring safety at 7T requires a multidisciplinary team of physicists, radiologists, and technologists knowledgeable of the practical and theoretic challenges accompanying this significant increase in magnetic field strength and hence Larmor frequency. This 7T safety team should develop local institutional safety policies and procedures, and ensure they remain current with this rapidly changing field. This group should perform risk/benefit analyses for individual cases as required, which is particularly relevant at 7T given the dearth of manufacturer certification of magnetic resonance conditionality for implanted devices.

Staff Training

Staff training is an important consideration when moving to 7T. Technologists need to be aware of strategies to minimize the incidence of dizziness and vertigo in patients on entering and exiting the scanner, by enforcing slow head movements in the vicinity of the magnet bore and ensuring correct positioning on the table. Such strategies are also essential for minimizing staff occupational exposure. The rapid removal of the patient table from the magnet in the event of an emergency will likely induce nausea in patients. The lack of vertical table movement and inability to undock the table on the current generation of 7T systems create further logistical challenges. Patient positioning within the 7T RF coils can impact significantly on image quality, and the use of dielectric pads requires careful consideration regarding their positioning (eg, to ensure their efficacious use and to avoid areas of low blood perfusion such as the eyes). Many conductive objects that are imaged as a matter of routine at 3T may be unsafe to image at 7T. Consequently, the safe prescreening of patients at 7T requires particular attention to the presence of conductive objects, whether implanted devices or nonremovable jewelry and tattoos. The current regulatory cleared 7T system imposes a minimum patient/subject weight of 30 kg, with implications for imaging small children. It is not advised to allow parents of young children to stand close to the magnet bore opening because of the potential for vestibulopathy and nausea in the attending parent. The scanning of patients with thermoregulatory compromise should also be carefully considered, while there are no data on the safety of imaging during pregnancy.

Many items of ancillary electronic equipment typically used in Zone 4, such as contrast injector pumps, physiologic monitoring systems, pumps, and anesthesia machines, have not been tested for safety at 7T, and introducing these into the Zone 4 requires careful assessment for potential unsafe magnetic forces. If a safe operating location is determined, it is recommended that such items be tethered securely to ensure they cannot be moved closer to the magnet, and staff should be trained accordingly in their use. Similar safety assessments should be carried out for passive devices such as gurneys, tables, and step stands where no prior information is available.

Radiologists should be aware of the different image characteristics at 7T to mitigate safety concerns relating to the potential for misdiagnoses. These include image contrast changes in many pulse sequences and image artifacts not typically encountered at lower field strengths or present with greater severity. These artifacts arise typically from nonuniform flip angle distributions, increased magnetic susceptibility effects, and pronounced signal drop-off in certain anatomic areas. Strategies to minimize such effects have been described,[45] and on-going developments, particularly in parallel transmit technology, are further demonstrating significant improvements in this area. Nevertheless, quantitative techniques such as whole-brain volumetrics require validation to ensure measurement accuracy is not compromised by artifacts such as geometric distortions, signal nonuniformity and drop-out, and variable contrast. Several imaging pulse sequences are not yet optimized for use at 7T, but here again considerable efforts by the research community are closing the gap with 3T MR imaging.

SUMMARY

The install base of clinical 7T MR imaging systems is increasing rapidly following the regulatory clearance of this technology in 2017 for patient diagnostic imaging and likely regulatory clearance of systems from additional manufacturers in the near future. The creation of a 7T safety team is recommended; this team should develop and maintain institutional safety policies and procedures that adhere to best practice. Two forthcoming ISMRM white papers on 7T MR imaging safety[47] and safety testing of experimental RF hardware will provide further resources to the high-field community in using this technology in a safe and efficacious manner.

DISCLOSURE

The authors have nothing to disclose.

REFERENCES

1. Ladd ME, Bachert P, Meyerspeer M, et al. Pros and cons of ultra-high-field MRI/MRS for human application. Prog Nucl Magn Reson Spectrosc 2018;109: 1–50.
2. Kraff O, Quick HH. 7T: Physics, safety, and potential clinical applications. J Magn Reson Imaging 2017; 46(6):1573–89.
3. Yacoub E, Shmuel A, Pfeuffer J, et al. Imaging brain function in humans at 7 Tesla. Magn Reson Med 2001;45(4):588–94.
4. International Electrotechnical Commission (IEC), 2015. 60601-2-33 Medical Electrical Equipment - Part 2-33: Particular requirements for the basic safety and essential performance of magnetic resonance equipment for medical diagnosis, Edition 3.2. ISBN 978-2-8322-2743-5.
5. Woods T, Delfino J, Rajan S. Assessment of Magnetically Induced Displacement Force and Torque on Metal Alloys Used in Medical Devices. ASTM International, doi: 10.1520/JTE20190096. Journal of Testing and Evaluation 2019.
6. Panych LP, Madore B. The physics of MRI safety. J Magn Reson Imaging 2018;47(1):28–43.
7. Grace Medical Inc. Magnetic Resonance Imaging (MRI) Information for Grace Medical otologic implants. Available at: http://www.gracemedical.com/mri-info/. Accessed January 8, 2020.

8. Kurz Medical Inc. MR information. Available at: https://www.kurzmed.com/en/certificates?file=files/media/MR-Information/MR_Information_en_Rev_06.pdf. Accessed January 8, 2020.

9. Novatech. Titanium Tracheal Support for Tracheopexy. Available at: https://www.novatech.fr/nc/en/ent-products/novatechr-tts.html?cid=3328&did=2407&sechash=00d0303c. Accessed January 8, 2020.

10. Glaukos Corp. iStent inject trabecular micro-bypass system. Available at: https://www.glaukos.com/wp-content/uploads/2016/05/45-0119-Rev-2-FINAL-ARTWORK-G2-M-IS-AS-IFU-vendor.pdf. Accessed January 8, 2020.

11. Wezel J, Kooij BJ, Webb AG. Assessing the MR compatibility of dental retainer wires at 7 Tesla. Magn Reson Med 2014;72(4):1191–8.

12. Oriso K, Kobayashi T, Sasaki M, et al. Impact of the static and radiofrequency magnetic fields produced by a 7T MR imager on metallic dental materials. Magn Reson Med Sci 2016;15(1):26–33.

13. Feng DX, McCauley JP, Morgan-Curtis FK, et al. Evaluation of 39 medical implants at 7.0 T. Br J Radiol 2015;88(1056):20150633.

14. Noureddine Y, Bitz AK, Ladd ME, et al. Experience with magnetic resonance imaging of human subjects with passive implants and tattoos at 7 T: a retrospective study. MAGMA 2015;28(6):577–90.

15. Chen B, Schoemberg T, Kraff O, et al. Cranial fixation plates in cerebral magnetic resonance imaging: a 3 and 7 Tesla in vivo image quality study. MAGMA 2016;29(3):389–98.

16. Thelen A, Bauknecht HC, Asbach P, et al. Behavior of metal implants used in ENT surgery in 7 Tesla magnetic resonance imaging. Eur Arch Otorhinolaryngol 2006;263(10):900–5.

17. Rauschenberg J, Groebner J, Semmier W, et al. How safe are intrauterine devices at MRI procedures with field strengths beyond 1.5T? Proceedings of the 19th ISMRM meeting. Montreal, May 6-13, 2011.

18. Ansems J, van der Kolk AG, Kroeze H, et al. MR Imaging of patients with stents is safe at 7.0 Tesla. Proceedings of the 20th ISMRM meeting. Melbourne, May 5-11, 2012.

19. Dula AN, Virostko J, Shellock FG. Assessment of MRI issues at 7 T for 28 implants and other objects. AJR Am J Roentgenol 2014;202(2):401–5.

20. Wrede KH, Chen B, Sure U, et al. Safety and Function of Programmable Ventriculo-Peritoneal Shunt Valves: An in vitro 7 Tesla Magnetic Resonance Imaging Study. Proceedings of the 25th ISMRM meeting. Honolulu, April 22-27, 2017.

21. Winkler SA, Alejski A, Wade T, et al. On the accurate analysis of vibroacoustics in head insert gradient coils. Magn Reson Med 2017;78(4):1635–45.

22. Fatahi M, Reddig A, Vijayalaxmi, et al. DNA double-strand breaks and micronuclei in human blood lymphocytes after repeated whole body exposures to 7T Magnetic Resonance Imaging. Neuroimage 2016;133:288–93.

23. Hansson B, Höglund P, Markenroth Bloch K, et al. Short-term effects experienced during examinations in an actively shielded 7 T MR. Bioelectromagnetics 2019;40(4):234–49.

24. Theysohn JM, Kraff O, Eilers K, et al. Vestibular effects of a 7 Tesla MRI examination compared to 1.5 T and 0 T in healthy volunteers. PLoS One 2014;9(3):e92104.

25. Rauschenberg J, Nagel AM, Ladd SC, et al. Multicenter study of subjective acceptance during magnetic resonance imaging at 7 and 9.4 T. Invest Radiol 2014;49(5):249–59.

26. Ward BK, Otero-Millan J, Jareonsettasin P, et al. Magnetic vestibular stimulation (MVS) as a technique for understanding the normal and diseased labyrinth. Front Neurol 2017;8:122.

27. Raaijmakers AJ, Italiaander M, Voogt IJ, et al. The fractionated dipole antenna: A new antenna for body imaging at 7 Tesla. Magn Reson Med 2016; 75(3):1366–74.

28. Erturk MA, Raaijmakers AJ, Adriany G, et al. A 16-channel combined loop-dipole transceiver array for 7 Tesla body MRI. Magn Reson Med 2017;77(2):884–94.

29. Raaijmakers AJ, Luijten PR, van den Berg CA. Dipole antennas for ultrahigh-field body imaging: a comparison with loop coils. NMR Biomed 2016; 29(9):1122–30.

30. Ipek O, Raaijmakers AJ, Lagendijk JJ, et al. Inter-subject local SAR variation for 7T prostate MR imaging with an eight-channel single-side adapted dipole antenna array. Magn Reson Med 2014;71(4):1559–67.

31. Gosselin MC, Neufeld E, Moser H, et al. Development of a new generation of high-resolution anatomical models for medical device evaluation: the Virtual Population 3.0. Phys Med Biol 2014;59(18):5287–303.

32. Eichfelder G, Gebhardt M. Local specific absorption rate control for parallel transmission by virtual observation points. Magn Reson Med 2011;66(5):1468–76.

33. Lee J, Gebhardt M, Wald LL, et al. Local SAR in parallel transmission pulse design. Magn Reson Med 2012;67(6):1566–78.

34. Kraff O, Wrede KH, Schoemberg T, et al. MR safety assessment of potential RF heating from cranial fixation plates at 7 T. Med Phys 2013;40(4):042302.

35. Sammet CL, Yang X, Wassenaar PA, et al. RF-related heating assessment of extracranial neurosurgical implants at 7T. Magn Reson Imaging 2013; 31(6):1029–34.

36. Winter L, Oberacker E, Ozerdem C, et al. On the RF heating of coronary stents at 7.0 Tesla MRI. Magn Reson Med 2015;74(4):999–1010.

37. Santoro D, Winter L, Muller A, et al. Detailing radio frequency heating induced by coronary stents: a 7.0 Tesla magnetic resonance study. PLoS One 2012;7(11):e49963.

38. Noureddine Y, Kraff O, Ladd ME, et al. In vitro and in silico assessment of RF-induced heating around intracranial aneurysm clips at 7 Tesla. Magn Reson Med 2018;79(1):568–81.

39. Ibrahim TS, Tang L, Kangarlu A, et al. Electromagnetic and modeling analyses of an implanted device at 3 and 7 Tesla. J Magn Reson Imaging 2007;26(5):1362–7.

40. Sammet S, Koch RM, Murrey DA, et al. MR-safety and compatibility of intrauterine devices at 3T and 7T. Proceedings of the 15th ISMRM meeting. Berlin, May 18-25, 2007.

41. Angelone LM, Vasios CE, Wiggins G, et al. On the effect of resistive EEG electrodes and leads during 7 T MRI: simulation and temperature measurement studies. Magn Reson Imaging 2006;24(6):801–12.

42. Brunner DO, De Zanche N, Frohlich J, et al. Travelling-wave nuclear magnetic resonance. Nature 2009;457(7232):994–8.

43. Teeuwisse WM, Brink WM, Haines KN, et al. Simulations of high permittivity materials for 7 T neuroimaging and evaluation of a new barium titanate-based dielectric. Magn Reson Med 2012;67(4):912–8.

44. O'Brien KR, Magill AW, Delacoste J, et al. Dielectric pads and low- B1+ adiabatic pulses: complementary techniques to optimize structural T1 w whole-brain MP2RAGE scans at 7 tesla. J Magn Reson Imaging 2014;40(4):804–12.

45. Fagan AJ, Welker KM, Amrami KK, et al. Image artifact management for clinical magnetic resonance imaging on a 7 T scanner using single-channel radiofrequency transmit mode. Invest Radiol 2019;54(12):781–91.

46. Vaidya MV, Lazar M, Deniz CM, et al. Improved detection of fMRI activation in the cerebellum at 7T with dielectric pads extending the imaging region of a commercial head coil. J Magn Reson Imaging 2018;48(2):431–40.

47. Fagan AJ, Bitz AK, Björkman-Burtscher IM, et al. 7T MR Safety. Journal of Magnetic Resonance Imaging. in print, 2020. doi:10.1002/jmri.27319.

MR Imaging Safety in the Interventional Environment

Bharathi D. Jagadeesan, MD

KEYWORDS

- Intraoperative MR imaging • MR-guided neurosurgery • MR-guided tumor resection • MRgFUS
- MR-guided interstitial laser ablation

KEY POINTS

- The safe and effective implementation of MR-guided techniques requires expertise in planning, equipment selection, zoning and installation of equipment, availability of safety personnel and medical directors, training for surgical personnel, contingency planning, and continuous implementation of emerging regulations.
- Appropriate selection of imaging, anesthesia and surgical equipment is key to ensuring safety with the interventional MR imaging system.
- All personnel involved in the routine operation and maintenance of the interventional MR imaging suite should undergo training as determined by institutional guidelines, testing, and continuous education regarding MR imaging safety.

INTRODUCTION

In the last 2 decades, a number of MR imaging–guided interventional procedures have established themselves, including MR imaging–guided neurosurgery, MR imaging–guided breast tissue biopsy, MR-guided focused ultrasound examination, and MR-guided robotic surgery.[1–4] The safe and effective implementation of these MR-guided techniques requires expertise in planning, equipment selection, zoning and installation of equipment, availability of safety personnel and medical directors, training for surgical personnel, contingency planning, and continuous implementation of emerging regulations. The safety concerns involved with MR-guided interventions, can be thought of as consisting of 2 distinct entities, that is, (a) safety concerns that are common to all diagnostic MR imaging equipment and (b) safety concerns that are unique to the interventional MR imaging milieu. These safety concerns are pertinent to the operators, patients, maintenance and service personnel, and indeed anyone who is likely to be involved in the upkeep and use of the interventional MR imaging suite. Herein, we review the requirements for the safe operation of interventional MR imaging suites in a systematic manner.

PLANNING AND BUILDING FOR INTERVENTIONAL MR IMAGING

Proper siting, zoning, and access control methods that promote safe use of the interventional MR imaging suite can be achieved with optimal planning.[5–7] Siting an interventional MR imaging system within the imaging department might mitigate the need for separate MR imaging zoning requirements, and as well as help with the ready availability of trained MR imaging personnel.[8] However, this is often impractical because of the distance between imaging departments and

Radiology, Neurology and Neurosurgery, University of Minnesota, MMC 292, Mayo Memorial Building, 420 Delaware Street SE, Minneapolis, MN 55455, USA
E-mail address: jagad002@umn.edu

Magn Reson Imaging Clin N Am 28 (2020) 583–591
https://doi.org/10.1016/j.mric.2020.07.007
1064-9689/20/© 2020 Elsevier Inc. All rights reserved.

surgical suites, operating room (OR) workflow issues, as well as the necessity to maintain a sterile environment and complex OR ventilation needs. Therefore, most interventional MR imaging systems tend to be situated within OR complexes. In this situation, the safe operation of interventional MR imaging systems can be enhanced by siting them at the end of a row of ORs, which minimizes the amount of foot traffic from personnel going in and out of other ORs, and clearly marking MR safety zones as required. The physical delineation of the 5 Gauss field strength limit, along the floor as well as ceiling of the OR are also helpful reminders to interventional MR imaging personnel.[9–11] Likewise, limiting access to the interventional MR imaging suite through doors that are clearly within the line of sight of the interventional MR imaging operators can avoid undetected entry of MR unsafe equipment or untrained personnel into the suite. Limiting access to the suite via personal identification systems capable of unlocking the doors will also enhance safety. Additionally, a prominent display of notifications outside the interventional suite doors, explicitly stating that the MR imaging is always on can be helpful. Some of these steps might require modification, depending on the whether the MR imaging system is a mobile construct that can traverse between multiple ORs, or if the MR imaging system remains stationary while patients from multiple ORs are transported in and out of the interventional MR imaging suite. Several successful floor plans and designs are widely available and could be followed in collaboration with the vendors.[8,10,12] One such plan at our institution incorporates an MR imaging that can be between 2 ORs, or parked at the center, allowing for an angiographic biplane table to be moved into the magnet bore (**Fig. 1**). This plan exploits the advantages of a mobile MR imaging (**Fig. 2**) while retaining the option for patient transport from the angiography suite into the magnet when it is in a stationary position in-between the 2 ORs, as well as the use of the MR imaging system for purely diagnostic imaging.

ZONING FOR THE INTERVENTIONAL MR IMAGING SUITE

Zone I and zone II designations are similar to zoning for diagnostic systems. However, zone III should include the substerile corridor and support space outside the scanner room.[11,13] Ideally, only MR conditional ventilators, and so on, should be stored in zone III to avoid accidental transport of MR unsafe equipment to an area within the 5 Gauss line. MR conditional or MR unsafe tools may need to be stored peripheral to a clearly

marked 5 Gauss line in many interventional settings, with physical tethering providing an important safety measure when practicable. The ORs wherein interventional MR imaging procedures are performed should be designated as zone IV (where the interventional MR imaging moves into the OR, or where there is no physical door between the OR and the interventional MR imaging scanner) or as zone III (when the patient is physically transported to the MR suite from the OR, provided that the door is shut between the 2 rooms). The 5 Gauss line must be contained within the OR in each of the ORs to which a mobile interventional MR imaging construct can be moved or it should be contained within the MR room for stationary interventional MR imaging units.

EQUIPMENT

Appropriate selection of imaging, anesthesia, and surgical equipment is key to ensuring safety with the interventional MR imaging system.

The specific static magnetic field strength of the interventional MR imaging system has major influences on other decisions related to the suite.[14,15] In addition, the available gradient strengths, slew rates, and gradient switching times are also factors that affect decisions regarding the purchase of interventional MR imaging equipment. The MR conditional designations for surgical equipment and prior implants will obviously differ when considering different field strengths. For higher field strength actively shielded interventional MR imaging systems, it is also very important to know that there will be a steeper change in the magnetic field gradient as the operator approaches the magnet bore when compared with a similar situation with lower field strength systems (the fringe fields might still resemble those encountered with lower field strength systems).[16] Greater B0 field inhomogeneities are associated with higher field strength interventional MR imaging systems with a greater potential for image distortion.[17,18] B0 inhomogeneities arising from fluctuations in power supply and thermal instability can be of greater consequence in high field strength interventional MR imaging systems and a provision should be made for backup power terminals. Additionally, image distortion from changes in susceptibility during surgical intervention (for instance, postcraniotomy changes) is more likely with higher field strength interventional MR imaging systems.[10] Image distortion also varies between different interventional MR imaging sequences for any given field strength, and this can affect surgical accuracy, outcome and patient safety.[19,20] The specific absorption rates also vary

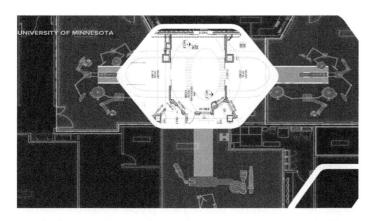

Fig. 1. Schematic showing the layout of a "T" suite consisting of 2 ORs with an interventional MR imaging parking bay at the center (inset shows an expanded view). The interventional MR imaging system moves from side to side to access either OR. The stem of the "T" leads to a biplane angiography suite. When the interventional MR imaging magnet is parked at the bay, the biplane angiography bed can be transported to the MR suite.

between different sequences for any given field strength. To address some of these issues, ultra-low field strength systems have been developed and deployed. These systems permit the use of an expanded array of MR imaging conditional surgical instruments, increasing operator comfort and with potential benefits to patient outcomes and safety.[21–23] This ability to accommodate more surgical instruments also makes it possible to perform a larger variety of interventional MR imaging procedures. However, ultralow field strength systems could lack some advanced functionality, such as diffusion tensor imaging, and the spatial resolution is less. The bore size of the interventional MR imaging system is best chosen in anticipation of the kinds of procedures that are likely to be performed in the interventional MR imaging suite. Performing procedures in excessively cramped conditions owing to small bore size in some systems could affect patient outcomes.

ANESTHESIA

Many interventional MR imaging–guided procedures require general anesthesia. Safe induction of anesthesia and resuscitation are facilitated by having a dedicated induction room next to the interventional MR imaging suite, where MR-unsafe equipment such as defibrillators, peripheral nerve stimulators, or Dopplers can be stored. The physical proximity of this room to the interventional MR imaging suite enables rapid transportation of the patient outside zone IV for the purposes of resuscitation.[11,24–26] In the case of mobile interventional MR imaging units, the scanner can be moved out of the OR during induction and recovery. All pieces of equipment used for anesthesia, including the anesthesia machine, cart, endotracheal tubes, intravenous poles, oxygen tanks, infusion pumps, endotracheal stylets and body warmers should not be permitted in zone IV if MR unsafe, or permitted only if

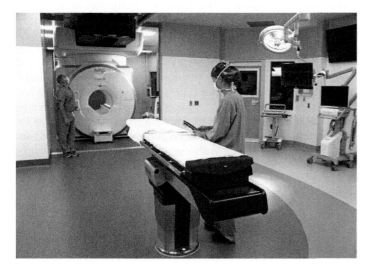

Fig. 2. OR table being readied in preparation for mobile interventional MR imaging system.

appropriate conditions are met related to their MR imaging conditional status. As is possible, material should be labeled depicting their MR safety classification as MR unsafe, conditional, or safe.[26,27]

The practice of general anesthesia in the interventional suite is influenced both by the magnetic field and by differences in patient positioning when compared with routine neurosurgical procedures. Most interventional MR imaging suites for neurosurgery have a head holder attached to the table; therefore, some patients may need to be placed prone and then pinned, making airway management more difficult, and increasing the risk for eye injury or cervical spine injury for the patient.[26,28] Additionally, an extended long ventilator circuit is necessary given the 160° to 180° turn of the patient. This factor poses specific challenges with pediatric intraoperative anesthesia in the interventional MR imaging suite owing to dead space concerns, and a minimum weight limit of 10 kg has been recommended for children undergoing interventional MR imaging procedures by some authors.[29] The length of the tubing and distance also make emergency airway management difficult for anesthetists, and particular attention must be paid to securing the endotracheal tube, or alternatively, nasotracheal intubation can be used.[30] Temperature maintenance is also more cumbersome in the interventional MR imaging setting, and small children and infants are particularly at risk for hypothermia.[31]

General anesthesia procedures require continuous monitoring of the patient's vital signs with electrocardiogram (ECG), pulse oximetry, arterial pressure monitoring, and so on. In the case of interventional MR imaging procedures performed under general anesthesia, artifacts can complicate ECG monitoring and pulse oximetry owing to electromagnetic interference from the scanner. This results in loss of integrity of the ECG waveform, which can be mitigated with available ECG filter systems. Even with the use of filtering techniques, the ECG waveforms are still likely to be altered and the anesthesia team must be very familiar with the end result ECG waveform, and also aware of whether a filter with or without T wave suppression is being used.[32] T wave amplitudes can be falsely elevated on ECG readings obtained in the interventional MR imaging suite from magnetohydrodynamic effects.[33] True lead I, II, and III waveforms may also not be obtainable.[34] Additionally, the electrical noise produced by anesthesia monitors can interfere with the performance of the interventional MR imaging system. The effects of electrical noise on imaging and vital signs monitoring equipment can be decreased with the use of portable extendable electrical noise shields that can be extended over the patient for imaging and retracted for surgery.[32] With respect to various leads and wires associated with vital signs monitoring equipment, closed loops, in which electrical currents are induced by the interventional MR imaging system, can be formed by wiring to skin contact, or looping/crossing of coils and wires with each other. Closed loops of electrical current can also arise from skin-to-skin contact, such as the crossing of limbs. The formation of conducting loops such as these can lead to thermal injuries from electrical currents. These injuries can be avoided by adequate padding and proper insulation. Alternatively, wireless ECG and pulse oximetry systems can be used.[25,26,35] Likewise, loops in fluid-containing intravenous lines should be avoided. With respect to neurosurgical procedures such as interventional MR imaging–guided brain tissue resections, motor or sensory evoked potential monitoring under general anesthesia can be challenging owing to potential heating of monitoring probes.[36–39]

SURGICAL INSTRUMENTS

It is highly recommended to use a checklist[37,38,40] for instrument screening and preparation before every procedure. All equipment should be counted before and after each procedure in the interventional MR imaging suite. An MR-safe instrument tray should be developed and standardized for each interventional MR imaging procedure. All surgical instruments used within zone IV must be MR safe or conditional and visible/trackable on MR imaging. MR conditional instruments can be considered as long as the parameters for conditional status are followed, and any artifacts are well-understood and anticipated. When the MR safety profile of an indispensable instrument is unknown, an MR safety evaluation by an experienced MR physicist can be helpful. This certification should follow the ASTM technical recommendations for the evaluation of MR-induced displacement forces (ASTM F2052-06), torque (ASTM F2213-06), and radiofrequency (RF)-induced heating (ASTM F2182-02).[41–43] It is prudent to have any essential equipment with ferromagnetic parts that could pose a projectile hazard tethered and bolted to the floor or walls outside the 5 Gauss line. The operators should be familiar with the materials used in interventional MR imaging surgical instrumentation, especially when repeat/corrective procedures are considered in the case of patients who may have previously had surgical implants placed elsewhere with or without interventional MR imaging guidance. In general, the most commonly used material for surgery, surgical steel, is unsafe with interventional MR imaging. However, instruments and implant hardware made of tantalum, titanium, nitinol, cobalt chromium, or precious metals are MR conditional and can be tolerated within the interventional MR imaging environment.[44,45]

The spatial resolution of the interventional MR imaging systems also needs to be considered when choosing surgical instruments that might be temporarily left in place within an organ such as cannulae or wire markers. Typically, these instruments are chosen to have some associated susceptibility artifact, which then enables their reliable detection even when they have small physical dimensions.[46,47] In the case of instruments that are made of diamagnetic material, those with enhanced MR imaging visibility secondary to the incorporation of small metallic markers, paramagnetic nanoparticles, inductively coupled single loops or self-resonant circuits within them, can be safely used in the interventional MR imaging environment.[48]

In the case of catheter-based interventions in the interventional MR imaging suite, or placement of deep brain stimulators or other procedures requiring the use of long wires, RF-induced heating poses a significant hazard from tissue injury secondary to localized high increases in the specific absorption rate, particularly from the use of RF intense sequences such as fast spin echo.[49] Maximal RF-induced heating is produced when the length of these instruments is a multiple of one-half the wavelength of the RF pulse. This usually translates to a length within the body of 25 to 30 cm in 1.5 T systems and about 10 to 13 cm for 3 T systems.[50] In the case of catheter-based interventional MR imaging procedures for the placement of vascular stents, the closed cell design of these stents acts as a faraday cage, precluding the detection of intraprocedural in-stent thrombosis.[51,52] Therefore, an alternative method such as intravascular ultrasound examination or angiography should be readily available to confirm the patency of these stents, or alternatively, stents with an integrated MR antenna can be used.

INTERVENTIONAL MR IMAGING SURGICAL ADJUNCTS AND THERAPEUTIC DEVICES
General Principles

The installation, maintenance, and operation of interventional MR imaging surgical adjuncts should be performed by properly screened and trained personnel at all times. An MR technologist or physicist should be present during these activities and ensure screening of these personnel. All adjunct instruments must be used in compliance with the vendor-issued instructions for use.

Interventional MR Robotic Surgical Systems

Interventional MR imaging robotic surgical tools can improve the outcome for interventional MR imaging–guided surgical procedures owing to the feasibility of intraoperative imaging without interruption of surgery because the robotic arms can be manipulated within the bore of the MR imaging device.[53] Robotic instrumentation can also decrease the number of operators within the interventional MR imaging suite. It is essential to identify MR imaging safe and MR conditional components for the robots for their safe operation; conditional components can be used within recommended parameters.

MR-Guided Focused Ultrasound Systems

MR-guided focused ultrasound systems use in the interventional MR imaging suite poses additional risks, such as skin burns on the side of the transducer owing to entrapped air between the skin and the transducer, especially with prolonged procedure times.[54,55] These burns are thought to occur from a combination of MR-related RF energy deposition and ultrasound energy.[15] Therefore, when MR-guided focused ultrasound systems are used, it is important to ensure an adequate seal between the patient's skin and the transducer to prevent burns. The measurement of skull density ratios for neurosurgical procedures and other similar tissue modeling techniques can be used for patient selection and MR-guided focused ultrasound systems.[56]

MR Imaging-Guided Interstitial Laser Ablation Systems

Special safety precautions pertaining to the use of a surgical laser need to be addressed when interventional MR imaging guidance is used for interstitial laser ablation. These precautions include placing "laser in use" signs outside the unit at all entrances and allowing only trained personnel to operate the laser.[57] It should also be remembered that, although the catheter and fiber used in the interstitial laser ablation system are MR imaging safe, other components of the laser system might only be MR conditional or MR unsafe. In some situations, the interstitial laser ablation workstation is sited in zone III, and the laser fiber is passed through a wave guide into zone IV on its way to the patient. Likewise, when a broken fiber is used with an interstitial laser ablation system, there is potential for patient or personnel injury as well as damage to the interventional MR system.[58,59] Protective glasses must be worn by the operators as protection in event of fiber breakage, and all material used in the interventional MR imaging suite should be fire resistant.[60]

PERSONNEL AND TRAINING

All personnel involved in the routine operation and maintenance of the interventional MR imaging suite should undergo training as determined by institutional guidelines, testing (online or written), and continuous education regarding MR imaging safety. Likewise, all personnel will need to undergo screening using the same criteria as for patients, particularly as relates to any implanted devices. Considerations regarding tattoos or other body adornments can be made on a case-by-case basis depending on the role of the individual and their expected proximity to the bore of the magnet. These operations should supervised by an MR imaging safety officer. Personnel should change into scrubs before entry into zone IV areas. All pagers, cell phones, clips, and any other ferromagnetic appliance or jewelry must be removed. Using scrubs without pockets can add an important additional layer of safety to guard against inadvertent transport of MR unsafe materials within the interventional MR imaging suite.

Occupational exposure to personnel who work regularly with the intraoperative MR imaging may also be considered. Currently, there are no recommended annual limits. When, operators are working in the interventional MR imaging suite, the International Commission on Non-ionizing Radiation Protection recommends that the change in magnetic flux density that the operators experience be kept below 2 T over a 3-second period. This strategy was prompted by concern over nausea and vertigo.[61,62] Rapid movement of the operators, particularly near the magnet bore, such as during emergency situations, could result in this threshold being exceeded. There is also the likelihood of visual disturbances owing to magneto phosphenes and peripheral nerve stimulation.[63–65] Some studies report that even static magnetic fields without movement can induce nausea.[66] Although specific instances of compromised safety for operators from nausea or magneto phosphenes have never been reported, it stands to reason that operator discomfort during sensitive procedures could potentially lead to avoidable errors.

In common with MR imaging in general, the acoustic noise produced by interventional MR imaging systems could also result in damage to hearing. Therefore, noise protection tools should be used by operators at all times when imaging is performed.

PATIENT SCREENING, PREPARATION, RESUSCITATION, AND TRANSPORT SAFETY SPECIFICS IN THE INTERVENTIONAL MR IMAGING SETTING

Interventional MR imaging–based surgical procedures should only be offered to patients who are known to benefit from such procedures or to patients participating in clinical trials that evaluate the usefulness of interventional MR imaging; and must be limited to institutional review board–approved studies. This principle is likely to decrease the risk to patients for whom the benefit of interventional MR imaging is questionable or unproven or is not under investigation. All patients who are considered eligible for interventional MR imaging–guided interventions should undergo the usual safety screening for MR imaging at the institution, in accordance with American College of Radiology guidelines.[9,13] The American College of Radiology aligns with guidance for performing MR imaging studies in patients with cardiac devices to the recommendations of the Heart Rhythm Society.[67]

All patients with implantable cardiac devices, including MR imaging-conditional and MR imaging nonconditional devices, must have their device properly programmed before MR imaging, and be closely monitored throughout the MR imaging examination by personnel trained in advanced cardiac life support.

After the screening of patients and approval for an interventional MR imaging procedure, all ferromagnetic material belonging to the patient must be removed in a manner that is analogous to the protocol for patients undergoing routine MR imaging. Subsequently, after the patient is transported to the interventional MR imaging suite, and before every interventional MR imaging procedure, a "FULL STOP AND FINAL CHECK" performed by the MR imaging technologist and support staff is specifically recommended by the American College of Radiology.[13] When positioning patients, direct skin-to-skin contact as well as crossing of limbs and so on, must be avoided to prevent the formation of closed conducting loops, which could result in burns. Likewise, patients should be gradually transported into the magnet bore to minimize the pull on implants from Lenz forces.[9,68] All leads to the patient should be insulated from contact with the skin. As described elsewhere in this article, leads and wires should not loop and should ideally run along the middle of the bore. All surgical drapes, gowns, towels, and other items that are used for the interventional MR imaging procedure should be free from increasingly commonly incorporated metals such as silver. There should be barrier measuring at least 1 cm in thickness between the transmission coil and the patient's skin surface.[13] The patients should be protected from acoustic noise, which depends on magnetic field strength as well as the sequences used.[15,69] Patients under anesthesia should also be protected from acoustic noise using noise protection systems. Intraoperative acute hemodynamic instability from arrythmias or blood loss or other factors can present a unique challenge during interventional MR imaging procedures. Patients might require acute resuscitation. All such acute resuscitation efforts should be performed after transporting the patient out of zone IV expeditiously. This practice will ensure that non–MR-safe equipment such as defibrillators, as well as the expertise of non–MR-trained essential personnel, are available to resuscitate the patient and eliminate the risk of projectile injuries. At the end of every procedure and after completion of any required postoperative imaging, an instrument count must once again be performed. The patient must be transported out of zone IV for postoperative recovery. Switching between MR safe and unsafe equipment (for instance, with vital sign monitors) to enable patient transport should happen outside zone IV. Finally, at the end of every interventional MR imaging procedure, standardized MR safe disinfection and cleaning practices must be followed.[13]

LEADERSHIP, MANAGEMENT, AND VIGILANCE

The operation of an interventional MR imaging suite is a complex undertaking involving specialists from multiple backgrounds, including surgeons, interventional radiologists, anesthesiologists, diagnostic radiologists, nurses, physicists, engineers, technologists, and maintenance personnel, all of whom share responsibility for patient and operator safety. In such a complex setting, safety can only be ensured by constituting a clear leadership structure with representation from all stake holders, and the vigilance of designated MR imaging safety officer(s). Clear and easily available protocols should be made available for training and screening of personnel. Accurate record keeping, regular meetings and consultation, a transparent feedback system, and prompt redressal of deficiencies are a must for patient safety. Additionally, all emerging evidence on MR imaging safety should be promptly incorporated into clinical operation of the interventional MR imaging suite. With such efforts, interventional MR imaging suites can be safely and successfully operated to improve the health of patients.

DISCLOSURE

The authors have nothing to disclose.

REFERENCES

1. Busse H, Kahn T, Moche M. Navigation Techniques for MRI-Guided Interventions. In: Kahn T, Busse H, editors. Interventional Magnetic Resonance Imaging. Medical Radiology. Berlin, Heidelberg: Springer; 2012. p. 53–75. https://doi.org/10.1007/174_2012_579.

2. Teichgräber UKM, Streitparth F, Güttler FV. High-Field Open MRI-Guided Interventions. In: Kahn T, Busse H, editors. Interventional Magnetic Resonance Imaging. Medical Radiology. Berlin, Heidelberg: Springer; 2012. p. 145–57. https://doi.org/10.1007/174_2012_618.

3. Lotz J. Interventional vascular MRI: moving forward. Eur Heart J 2012;34(5):327–9.

4. Hata N, Moreira P, Fischer G. Robotics in MRI-guided interventions. Top Magn Reson Imaging 2018;27(1):19–23.

5. Jankovski A, Francotte F, Vaz G, et al. Intraoperative magnetic resonance imaging at 3-T using a dual independent operating room-magnetic resonance imaging suite: development, feasibility, safety, and preliminary experience. Neurosurgery 2008;63(3):412–24.

6. Mittal S, Black PM. Intraoperative magnetic resonance imaging in neurosurgery: the Brigham concept. Acta Neurochir 2006;98:77–86.

7. Nour SG, Lewin JS. Creating a clinical interventional MRI service. Top Magn Reson Imaging 2018;27(1):25–31.

8. Azmi H, Gibbons M, DeVito MC, et al. The interventional magnetic resonance imaging suite: experience in the design, development, and implementation in a pre-existing radiology space and review of concepts. Surg Neurol Int 2019;10:101.

9. Expert Panel on MR Safety, Kanal E, Barkovich AJ, et al. ACR guidance document on MR safe practices: 2013. J Magn Reson Imaging 2013;37(3):501–30.

10. Kettenbach J, Kacher DF, Kanan AR, et al. Intraoperative and interventional MRI: recommendations for a safe environment. Minim Invasive Ther Allied Technol 2009;15(2):53–64.

11. Johnston T, Moser R, Moeller K, et al. Intraoperative MRI: safety. Neurosurg Clin N Am 2009;20(2):147–53.

12. Hall WA, Galicich W, Bergman T, et al. 3-Tesla intraoperative MR imaging for neurosurgery. J Neurooncol 2006;77(3):297–303.

13. ACR Committee on MR Safety, Greenberg TD, Hoff MN, et al. ACR guidance document on MR

safe practices: updates and critical information 2019. J Magn Reson Imaging 2020;51(2):331–8.

14. Truwit CL, Hall WA. Intraoperative magnetic resonance imaging-guided neurosurgery at 3-T. Neurosurgery 2006;58(suppl_4). ONS-338-ONS-346.

15. Kim SJ, Kim KA. Safety issues and updates under MR environments. Eur J Radiol 2017;89:7–13.

16. Derakhshan JJ, Duerk JL. Update to pulse sequences for interventional MR Imaging. Magn Reson Imaging Clin N Am 2005;13(3):415–29.

17. Soher BJ, Dale BM, Merkle EM. A review of MR physics: 3T versus 1.5T. Magn Reson Imaging Clin N Am 2007;15(3):277–90.

18. Farahani K, Sinha U, Sinha S, et al. Effect of field strength on susceptibility artifacts in magnetic resonance imaging. Comput Med Imaging Graph 1990;14(6):409–13.

19. Tavares WM, Tustumi F, Leite CDC, et al. An image correction protocol to reduce distortion for 3-T stereotactic MRI. Neurosurgery 2014;74(1):121–7.

20. Baldwin LN, Wachowicz K, Thomas SD, et al. Characterization, prediction, and correction of geometric distortion in 3T MR images. Med Phys 2007;34(2):388–99.

21. Schulder M, Liang D, Carmel PW. Cranial surgery navigation aided by a compact intraoperative magnetic resonance imager. J Neurosurg 2001;94(6):936–45.

22. Schulder M, Carmel PW. Intraoperative magnetic resonance imaging: impact on brain tumor surgery. Cancer Control 2003;10(2):115–24.

23. Rubino GJ, Farahani K, McGill D, et al. Magnetic resonance imaging-guided neurosurgery in the magnetic fringe fields: the next step in neuronavigation. Neurosurgery 2000;46(3):643–54.

24. Hemingway M, Kilfoyle M. Safety planning for intraoperative magnetic resonance imaging. AORN J 2013;98(5):508–24.

25. Berkow LC. Anesthetic management and human factors in the intraoperative MRI environment. Curr Opin Anaesthesiol 2016;29(5):563–7.

26. Pal R, Maurtua M. Anesthetic challenges during neurosurgical procedures using intraoperative magnetic resonance imaging systems (IMRIS), literature review and case report. Br J Anaesth 2015;115(eLetters). https://doi.org/10.1093/bja/el_12174.

27. Tan TK, Goh J. The anaesthetist's role in the setting up of an intraoperative MR imaging facility. Singapore Med J 2009;50(1):4.

28. Edgcombe H, Carter K, Yarrow S. Anaesthesia in the prone position. Br J Anaesth 2008;100(2):165–83.

29. Roder C, Breitkopf M, Sotirios MS, et al. Beneficial impact of high-field intraoperative magnetic resonance imaging on the efficacy of pediatric low-grade glioma surgery. Neurosurg Focus 2016;40(3):E13.

30. McClain CD, Rockoff MA, Soriano SG. Anesthetic concerns for pediatric patients in an intraoperative MRI suite. Curr Opin Anaesthesiol 2011;24(5):480–6.

31. Bissonnette B. Temperature monitoring in pediatric anesthesia. Int Anesthesiol Clin 1992;30(4):63–76.

32. Dzwonczyk R, Fujii JT, Simonetti O, et al. Electrical noise in the intraoperative magnetic resonance imaging setting. Anesth Analg 2009;108(1):181–6.

33. Keltner JR, Roos MS, Brakeman PR, et al. Magnetohydrodynamics of blood flow. Magn Reson Med 1990;16(1):139–49.

34. Kanal E, Shellock FG. Patient monitoring during clinical MR imaging. Radiology 1992;185(3):623–9.

35. Tan TK, Goh J. The anesthetist's role in the setting up of an intra-operative imaging facility. Singapore Med J 2009;50(1):4.

36. Bottomley PA. Turning up the heat on MRI. J Am Coll Radiol 2008;5(7):853–5.

37. Sarnthein J, Lüchinger R, Piccirelli M, et al. Prevalence of complications in intraoperative magnetic resonance imaging combined with neurophysiologic monitoring. World Neurosurg 2016;93:168–74.

38. Wong JM, Bader AM, Laws ER, et al. Patterns in neurosurgical adverse events and proposed strategies for reduction. Neurosurg Focus 2012;33(5):E1.

39. Cherkashin M, Berezina N, Serov AL, et al. Safety management for MR-guided interventions. Investing Magn Reson Imaging 2016;20(3):152.

40. Stienen MN, Fierstra J, Pangalu A, et al. The Zurich checklist for safety in the intraoperative magnetic resonance imaging suite: technical note. Oper Neurosurg (Hagerstown) 2018;16(6):756–65.

41. ASTM. ASTM F2052-15, standard test method for measurement of magnetically induced displacement force on medical devices in the magnetic resonance environment. West Conshohocken (PA): ASTM International; 2015. Available at: www.astm.org.n.d.

42. ASTM. ASTM F2182-19e1, standard test method for measurement of radio frequency induced heating on or near passive implants during magnetic resonance imaging. West Conshohocken (PA): ASTM International; 2019. Available at: www.astm.org.n.d.

43. ASTM. ASTM F2213-17, standard test method for measurement of magnetically induced torque on medical devices in the magnetic resonance environment. West Conshohocken (PA): ASTM International; 2017. Available at: www.astm.org.n.d.

44. Melzer A, Michitsch ST, Konak S, et al. Nitinol in magnetic resonance imaging. Minim Invasive Ther Allied Technol 2004;13(4):261–71.

45. Shellock FG. Biomedical implants and devices: assessment of magnetic field interactions with a 3.0-Tesla MR system. J Magn Reson Imaging 2002;16(6):721–32.

46. Lewin JS, Duerk JL, Jain VR, et al. Needle localization in MR-guided biopsy and aspiration: effects of

field strength, sequence design, and magnetic field orientation. Am J Roentgenol 1996;166(6): 1337–45.

47. Melzer A, Schmidt AM, Kipfmüller K, et al. Prerequisites for magnetic resonance image-guided interventions and endoscopic surgery. Minim Invasive Ther Allied Technol 1996;5(3):255–62.

48. Kuehne T, Weiss S, Brinkert F, et al. Catheter visualization with resonant markers at MR imaging–guided deployment of endovascular stents in swine. Radiology 2004;233(3):774–80.

49. Nitz WR, Oppelt A, Renz W, et al. On the heating of linear conductive structures as guide wires and catheters in interventional MRI. J Magn Reson Imaging 2001;13(1):105–14.

50. Schick F. Whole-body MRI at high field: technical limits and clinical potential. Eur Radiol 2005;15(5): 946–59.

51. Teitelbaum GP, Bradley WG, Klein BD. MR imaging artifacts, ferromagnetism, and magnetic torque of intravascular filters, stents, and coils. Radiology 1988;166(3):657–64.

52. Klemm T, Duda S, Machann J, et al. MR imaging in the presence of vascular stents: a systematic assessment of artifacts for various stent orientations, sequence types, and field strengths. J Magn Reson Imaging 2000;12(4):606–15.

53. Guo Z, Leong MCW, Su H, et al. Techniques for stereotactic neurosurgery: beyond the frame, toward the intraoperative magnetic resonance imaging–guided and robot-assisted approaches. World Neurosurg 2018;116:77–87.

54. Joo B, Park MS, Lee SH, et al. Pain palliation in patients with bone metastases using magnetic resonance-guided focused ultrasound with conformal bone system: a preliminary report. Yonsei Med J 2015;56(2):503–9.

55. Zaher S, Gedroyc W, Lyons D, et al. A novel method to aid in the visualisation and treatment of uterine fibroids with MRgFUS in patients with abdominal scars. Eur J Radiol 2010;76(2):269–73.

56. D'Souza M, Chen KS, Rosenberg J, et al. Impact of skull density ratio on efficacy and safety of magnetic resonance–guided focused ultrasound treatment of essential tremor. J Neurosurg 2019;1–6. https://doi.org/10.3171/2019.2.jns183517.

57. Larson PS, Vadivelu S, Azmi-Ghadimi H, et al. Neurosurgical laser ablation and MR thermometry:

risks of multisite workflow pattern. J Healthc Risk Manag 2017;36(4):7–18.

58. Labo JA, Rogers ME. Can broken fiber optics produce hazardous laser beams? Proc. SPIE 1892, Medical Lasers and Systems II. Los Angeles (CA): SPIE; 1993. p. 176-87. https://dx.doi.org/10.1117/12.147498.

59. Absten GT, Sliney DH. Assessing the safety of broken Holmium laser fibers ILSC. Journal of Laser Applications 2015;1:228–34. https://doi.org/10.2351/1.5056842.

60. Wöllmer W, Schade G, Kessler G. Endotracheal tube fires still happen – A short overview. Medical Laser Application 2010;25(2):118–25.

61. ICNIRP. Guidelines for limiting exposure to electric fields induced by movement of the human body in a static magnetic field and by time-varying magnetic fields below 1 Hz. Health Phys 2014;106(3):418–25.

62. Gorlin A, Hoxworth JM, Mueller J. Occupational hazards of exposure to magnetic resonance imaging. Anesthesiology 2015;123(4):976–7.

63. Lövsund P, Oberg PA, Nilsson SE. Magneto- and electrophosphenes: a comparative study. Med Biol Eng Comput 1980;18(6):758–64.

64. Sammet S. Magnetic resonance safety. Abdom Radiol (NY) 2016;41(3):444–51.

65. Davids M, Guérin B, Vom Endt A, et al. Prediction of peripheral nerve stimulation thresholds of MRI gradient coils using coupled electromagnetic and neurodynamic simulations. Magnet Reson Med 2018;81(1):686–701.

66. van Rongen E, Saunders RD, van Deventer ET, et al. Static fields: biological effects and mechanisms relevant to exposure limits. Health Phys 2007;92(6):584–90.

67. Indik JH, Gimbel JR, Abe H, et al. 2017 HRS expert consensus statement on magnetic resonance imaging and radiation exposure in patients with cardiovascular implantable electronic devices. Heart Rhythm 2017;14(7):e97–153.

68. Kanal E, Barkovich AJ, Bell C, et al. ACR guidance document for safe MR practices: 2007. Am J Roentgenol 2007;188(6):1447–74.

69. Smith JA. Hazards, safety, and anesthetic considerations for magnetic resonance imaging. Top Companion Anim Med 2010;25(2):98–106.

MR Imaging Safety Events
Analysis and Improvement

Robert E. Watson Jr, MD, PhD[a],*, Mussie Tesfaldet, RT[b], Julee Warren, RT[a], Michael N. Hoff, PhD[b]

KEYWORDS

- MR imaging safety • MR imaging burns • MR imaging projectiles

KEY POINTS

- Contemporary MR imaging practices face increasing safety risks associated with tight patient scheduling, relative shortfalls in MR imaging technologist availability, complex implantable devices, and increasing MR imaging environment complexity.
- By analyzing MR imaging safety events with debriefings and root cause analyses, specific gaps and conditions that led to the events can be identified and provide a basis for improved policies and procedures to prevent similar incidents from occurring going forward.
- Recent revisions to the American College of Radiology Guidance document on safe MR practices propose improvements to standards of care that can decrease chances that incidents, similar to those described in this article, will occur.
- Standardization of MR imaging safety organization by appointing MR safety Medical Directors, MR Safety Officers, and MR Safety Experts can be expected to ensure best practices.

INTRODUCTION

There are many ongoing efforts to improve the state of MR safety. There have been substantial revisions to the American College of Radiology (ACR) MR safety guidance document and increasing efforts to standardize operational infrastructure around MR imaging safety with named individuals serving as MR Medical Directors (MRMDs), MR Safety Officers (MRSOs), and MR Safety Experts (MRSEs).[1] The American Board of Magnetic Resonance Safety now exists with the aim of credentialing individuals in these positions through role-specific examinations. Despite incremental gains in MR safety, many evolving challenges remain in the field that are related to increasingly fast MR imaging workflow and time pressure, complex and evolving information sources including electronic medical records, frequent MR imaging technologist staff shortages associated with rapid MR imaging practice growth and a competitive job market,[2] complicated patients with ever-increasing numbers of implanted devices, as well as increasingly complex intraoperative and hybrid procedural practices.

As detailed in this article, multiple factors associated with contemporary clinical MR imaging create distinct patient and MR imaging personnel safety risks. There is great awareness in the MR imaging community of the need to improve MR imaging safety practices.[3] Strong attractive forces associated with the main magnetic field create the possibility of dangerous projectile incidents if ferromagnetic objects are inadvertently allowed to enter into Zone IV. Because of the spatial gradient magnetic field,[4] an unsuspecting individual transporting a ferromagnetic object may initially detect virtually no force on the object until it is suddenly and forcefully drawn toward the magnet. Time-varying gradient magnetic fields

[a] Department of Radiology, Mayo Clinic, 200 First Street Southwest, Rochester, MN 55905, USA; [b] Department of Radiology, University of Washington, 1959 Northeast Pacific Street, Seattle, WA 98195, USA
* Corresponding author.
E-mail address: watson.robert16@mayo.edu

Magn Reson Imaging Clin N Am 28 (2020) 593–600
https://doi.org/10.1016/j.mric.2020.07.004
1064-9689/20/© 2020 Elsevier Inc. All rights reserved.

and radiofrequency (RF) magnetic fields can interact with implanted or on-planted devices and result in patient harm if not correctly recognized and accounted for. RF fields can also cause burns, which may be exacerbated by poor patient positioning or MR unsafe patient garments, jewelry, and other adornments.

In an effort to learn from past MR safety events,[5] this report describes several MR imaging safety incidents from the authors' institutions. Contributing factors are detailed, and responses to these incidents that strive for safer practices going forward are described. These illustrative cases are of interest to the MR imaging safety community, especially in the context of new recommendations included in the ACR MR imaging safety committee document on MR safety.[1] For other pertinent incidents, the most commonly reported patient safety events are reported to the Manufacturer and User Facility Device Experience (MAUDE) database.[6]

Avoid Zone IV Doorway Ferromagnetic Object Breaches with a Barrier

Incident 1a

A wheelchair-bound, small-stature, low-weight outpatient child was to receive an MR imaging. The patient was changed into an MR imaging safe gown. The father wheeled the patient into Zone III in the patient's MR imaging unsafe wheelchair. The wheelchair was securely tethered to the wall with dedicated straps and clasps well away from the Zone IV door. The father, who was appropriately screened for MR imaging safety, was granted permission to stay with the child in Zone IV while the scan was being performed. The father carried the child from the tethered wheelchair to the docked MR imaging table. The scan was performed uneventfully. Although the technologist came into Zone IV at the conclusion of the study to attend to the child, the father, without being asked to do so, left Zone IV through the open door, untethered the wheelchair, and wheeled it back toward Zone IV. As he was crossing the threshold, the technologist noticed his presence and shouted for him to stop. A clinical assistant in the area heard this and guided the father and the wheelchair back to Zone III to retether it. An MR imaging conditional wheelchair was then used to remove the patient from Zone IV.

Incident 1b

A full-spine MR imaging examination was completed. The technologist entered Zone IV and began disconnecting monitoring leads from the patient. A second technologist was distracted by a physician phone call. At that time an emergency room float nurse entered the MR imaging room through the open door with an MR-unsafe stretcher for patient transfer. The technologist attending to the patient was facing away from the nurse and stretcher but on turning around noticed it. The technologist quickly pushed the stretcher out of the magnet room.

Incident 1c

An incarcerated patient was admitted for MR imaging. The patient was waiting to be scanned while on the MR imaging table in Zone IV as the scanning technologists were making phone calls to the radiologist for protocol-related queries. During this time the corrections officer responsible for the patient, equipped with a firearm, restraining devices, and various other metallic devices attached to his person, walked into Zone IV through the open door to talk to the patient. One of the technologists saw the officer in the room and quickly followed and requested that he step out of the room due to the various potential projectiles. The corrections officer stepped out of the MR imaging room and when queried admitted that he had been told not to enter but had forgotten. The patient was removed from Zone IV and overseen by the corrections officer in the Zone III area while the technologists completed their remaining tasks. The patient was then scanned and left the department without further incident. Multiple corrections officers, the covering physician, and family members of the prisoner were made aware of this near miss that could have had serious consequences.

Learning points Additional instances of less ferromagnetic materials crossing the Zone IV threshold through an open Zone IV door while attending to patients have occurred, all without injury. In the aforementioned scenarios, had any of the ferromagnetic objects become projectiles, there was substantial risk of significant injury or death. A common factor in these events was while attending to their duties, technologists left the Zone IV entry point open to free passage, without any physical barrier. As a result, the authors' institutions have implemented new departmental policies for ensuring that free access through the Zone IV entry point is always restricted. This entails that either the Zone IV door is closed, that a barrier such as a bright yellow retractable safety strap or plastic chain is affixed, or responsible level 2 personnel are physically stationed at the doorway. This, along with appropriate updates to MR imaging safety training, are essential to reduce the chances of unintentionally bringing unsafe ferromagnetic objects into Zone IV. A common scenario is that despite being told repeatedly not to enter Zone IV, non-MR imaging personnel in

Zone III frequently forget, and a physical barrier at the door can prevent entry.

Since this policy was enacted it has been well received by MR imaging staff and compliance has been excellent. There was initial concern that technologists and others would resist taking the time to close the door or deploy the strap, but this has not been the case, and MR imaging staff seem to appreciate the augmented safety margin that this practice provides. Importantly, the update to the ACR MR imaging safety committee document on MR safety has specifically recommended the following:[1]

Zone IV
The entry door to Zone IV (MR system room) should be closed except when it must be open for patient care or room/MR system maintenance. During the times that the door to the MR system room must remain open, a "caution" barrier is recommended at the entry to Zone IV to inhibit unintended passage of personnel and/or materials from Zone III to IV. Examples of caution barriers include easily adjusted straps or plastic chains secured across the scanner room doorway.

The institutions have also adjusted policy to ensure enhanced vigilance with regard to prisoners and corrections officers. As a preliminary measure, nonferrous restraining devices are requested of the corrections department for the MR imaging scan. Thorough MR screening of the patient and the accompanying correctional officer occurs in Zone II. All efforts to restrict ferrous materials from entering Zone III are made to avoid the possibility that they could become projectiles, and the officer is educated on this possibility with additional emphasis if the ferrous objects, including firearms, are absolutely essential in Zone III to maintain security. This conforms with recommendations in the update to the ACR MR imaging safety committee document on MR safety:[1]

Patient and Non-MR Personnel Screening
Guidance on the management of prisoners with restraints undergoing MR examinations has also been previously detailed.[7–10] However, guidance on prison or security personnel weapons (ie, firearms) has not been previously mentioned. Ferromagnetic firearm weapons should not be permitted into Zone III unless deemed absolutely essential for maintenance of security due to the design of the facility. Furthermore, ferromagnetic firearms that are loaded pose a serious threat in Zone IV (the MR system room) due to the possibility of inadvertent discharge.[11]

A Full-Stop/Final Check at the Zone IV Door Can Ensure Unwanted Metals Are Restricted Access

Incident 2a

A patient was brought from the emergency room with a leg in traction for an MR imaging scan. Orthopedics was called to remove the traction device from the patient before entry in Zone IV. The apparatus that hooks to the Steinman Pin was removed from the patient, wrapped in a towel, and left within blankets between the patient's legs. The admitting technologist did not notice this apparatus as the patient was brought into Zone IV. The patient was positioned on the MR imaging table, and when brought toward the scanner, the device was pulled from the blankets toward magnet, striking the patient's perineal area before becoming affixed to the magnet. The patient was not significantly injured.

Incident 2b

An intubated inpatient was transported from the emergency department to MR imaging room for a brain scan. Multiple staff in Zone III, including nurses, technologists, assistants, and an interpreter in Zone III engendered a complicated patient preparation scenario. In the process of screening and bringing the patient into Zone IV, an MR imaging unsafe intravenous (IV) pole was brought into the scan room by an MR imaging technologist. The pole was pulled away from the technologist and patient toward the magnet, becoming affixed to the magnet bore. The lines from the IV pole were carefully removed from the pole, and the patient was removed from the scan room safely. The patient was unharmed. The magnetic field needed to be ramped down by vendor service engineers until the pole could be safely removed from Zone IV.

Incident 2c

An interventional MR imaging site has a 3T magnet MR imaging separated by laterally sliding doors from an operating room (OR). In addition to laser ablation and focused ultrasound cases, the site is used frequently to assess for extent of tumor resection. Patients are MR scanned with the surgical wounds still open, and the patient may return to OR if imaging demonstrates subtotal resection.

One complex tumor resection case lasted in excess of 12 hours. The patient was being readied for transfer to MR imaging to assess extent of tumor resection. Some personnel had left for the day, including those associated with electromyography (EMG) monitoring of the patient. Leads attached to the patient that are normally removed by the EMG personnel had remained in place. A certified registered nurse anesthetist (CRNA), working well beyond normal working hours, assisted by finding a pair of small scissors and cutting the leads near the patient's skin surface. The patient was prepared for transfer into Zone IV by OR staff, and a time-out, controlled by a level 2 technologist serving as the MRSO, was performed on the CRNA before crossing the threshold into Zone IV. All pockets were patted down and the CRNA was deemed safe to proceed. The CRNA was wheeling anesthesia equipment into Zone IV ahead of the patient, and it was at this time that a projectile was seen flying into the bore of the magnet. The CRNA and MRSO found the small scissors in the bore, and with considerable effort, pulled them off the bore and walked them out of the room, well away from the patient and other personnel. The patient was then scanned uneventfully and returned to the OR for wound closure.

Root cause analysis revealed that the CRNA had mistakenly placed the scissors in a top front pocket of their scrubs, behind folded papers with patient notes. The pocket was patted down during the time out before crossing the threshold into Zone IV, but due to the papers in front of the scissors, the scissors were not detected.

Learning points These 3 events shared the common theme of projectile events occurring in the context of scanning complex, nonroutine patients. Evolving and improving MR imaging safety practices, along with awareness of the significantly increased risks in such scenarios, can be anticipated to lessen the chances of similar incidents going forward. Although MR imaging personnel clearly understand the risks of unsafe ferromagnetic materials entering Zone IV, and generally are excellent at screening for such unsafe items, in complex situations, safety gaps can occur. For this reason, strict procedures and checklists should be implemented and adhered to. In especially challenging scenarios, as in intraoperative MR imaging settings, and in hybrid procedural suites, identifying a designated MRSO as the point person whose role it is to ensure safety of the team and the patient should be strongly considered. This can address distractions and unusual circumstances that could derail MR safety efforts if not approached in a systematic manner.

The updated ACR guidance document on MR safe practice now recommends that there be a "full-stop and final check" before patients, staff, and equipment can access Zone IV.[1] This states:

Full-Stop and Final Check
Some instances where the patient is sedated or anesthetized, an inpatient, or an emergent case, a "full-stop and final check" performed by the MR imaging technologist along with support staff is recommended to confirm the completion of MR safety screening for the patient, support equipment, and personnel MR screening immediately prior to crossing from Zone III to Zone IV. "Full-stop and final check" may also be useful for non-sedated outpatients and inpatients prior to movement from Zone III to Zone IV. The purpose of this final check is to confirm patient name, ensure that all screening has been appropriately performed, and that there has been no change in patient and/or equipment status while in Zone III.

In addition to the full-stop and final check, extensive testing of any equipment in the MR environment and appropriate MR safety labeling should be performed. Any materials needed that are MR imaging unsafe, such as the IV pole in case 2b, should be removed from the department and replaced with MR imaging safe or conditional ones.

The intraoperative MR imaging environment requires constant assessment to identify additional essential safety measures. MR imaging personnel now wear pocketless scrubs. Ferromagnetic detector screening of personnel traversing from Zone III to IV has been implemented. For excessively long surgical cases, if the neurosurgeon does not expect to resect additional tumor, regardless of what an MR imaging would show, MR imaging is being deferred until the next day to minimize chances that fatigue could play a contributory role in an MR imaging safety incident.

Finally, in situations where ferromagnetic material is affixed to the bore, special safety considerations should be undertaken before attempts to remove the object. Moving a ferromagnetic object across the rapidly changing spatial magnetic gradient field near the opening of the magnet bore can cause unpredictable torque and force on an object. This creates a risk that the object may break free from the individual's grasp and become a dangerous projectile *once again*, with risk of injury to personnel or a patient in proximity. At the authors' institutions, MR imaging service personnel are consulted in such a situation and they handle rare removal of ferromagnetic objects from the bore.

Appropriate Transmit Coil Insulation Is Essential to Avoid RadiofrequencyRF Burns

Incident 3a
An outpatient was to receive an elbow MR imaging examination. The patient had a prosthetic leg

and was wearing athletic stretch leggings. The medical assistant (MA) directed the patient to a changing room to remove all clothing and put on a gown, per protocol. Patient changed as directed but did not remove the athletic leggings. The MR imaging technologist and MA brought the patient into the examination room to be positioned for the elbow examination following safety screening. It became clear later that the patient's lower back was in proximity to the bore with apparently only a bedsheet between the patient and the bore. The scan commenced, and the scanning MR imaging technologist handed off the case to another technologist midway through the case. The patient was verbally checked 3 times during the examination without reported issue. The patient began to move toward the end of the last MR imaging sequence and mentioned that it was warm, but the technologist did not hear this. The technologist asked the patient to keep still, stating that it was almost over. Patient complied and, again, never mentioned warmth or discomfort. When the technologist came to remove the patient from the scanner, the patient was sweaty and mentioned a burning sensation perceived as friction around the upper margin of the leggings that had caused motion during the scan. The supervising technologist was alerted, and a radiology nurse and fellow determined the area of warmth to be a burn posterior to the patient's left hip. A follow-up visit was arranged by the MRMD for the patient to be examined by a dermatologist. It was not clear if the leggings contained metallic fibers potentially contributing to the burn or if the mechanism was solely a result of proximity to the bore, being separated only by the sheet.

Incidents 3b

Several additional skin burns have occurred in a similar fashion to the one described in incident 3a related to improper pad positioning. Notably, in one case, a burn resulted despite proper positioning of a pad that was subsequently found to be worn out, permitting skin to be in unsafe proximity to the bore wall.

Learning points Burns are the single most common adverse event reported to the Food and Drug Administration MAUDE database,[6] and there are many actions that should be followed to avoid their occurrence. For most MR imaging examinations, the transmitting RF coil is housed within the magnet bore and can induce electrical currents in any conductive substance nearby. Excessive heating can occur in subcutaneous fat, where there is a relative paucity of pain

receptors, such that significant burns may be evolving before being detected by the patient. There are even greater risks in the setting of anesthetized patients who cannot sense a burn in progress. The patient should be separated from contact or proximity with the magnet bore with an appropriately thick layer of padding to prevent burns, as discussed in the updated ACR guidance document on MR safe practices:[1]

Burn Prevention
To help safeguard against thermal injuries or burns, insulating pads should be placed between the patient's skin and any transmit RF coil located behind the walls and ceiling of the bore of the magnet system, especially the area of the transmit RF body coil, to ensure spacing between the bore wall and the patient's skin. A single-layer bed sheet is insufficient insulation or spacing. It is also important to recognize that large conducting loops may be created within the patient's own tissues by points of skin-to-skin contact, such as thigh-to-thigh contact. Thus, providing insulation in such areas may also be required to prevent burns. To prevent excessive heating and possible burns in patients in association with MR procedures, the previously published guidelines are recommended.[12]

Also, in an effort to prevent patient burns, it is essential that patients remove clothing and be fully gowned before entry into Zone IV due to the increasing prevalence of metallic fibers in clothing.[13] The updated ACR guidance document on MR safe practices now makes explicit gowning recommendations that warn about new synthetic types of clothing that use metallic thread:[1]

Patient and Non-MR Personnel Screening
Some materials used in clothing have been increasingly associated with thermal injury and/or burns in patient's undergoing MR imaging. Additionally, recent trends in the manufacturing of clothing and other related products have incorporated ferromagnetic and/or conductive materials (eg, antimicrobial silver and copper) that are not reliably disclosed in labeling.[13] Such clothing products include, but are not limited to, sportswear (including underwear), brassieres, orthotic-related items (eg, stump covers or stump shrinkers), and blankets.[14] Reliance on clothing labeling is not sufficient, as the Federal Trade Commission (FTC) "guidelines"

allow clothing to contain as much as 5% impurities, which could be significant for a patient undergoing an MR imaging examination.[15] For areas in or around the volume of transmitted RF power, we recommend patients wear only MR-Safe gowns or scrubs supplied by the imaging facility.

Screening Considerations and Potential Utility of Ferromagnetic Detection

Incident 4a

A research subject reported to MR imaging mid-morning for a noncontrast head scan. Before reporting, there was awareness of an implanted and inflatable penile prosthesis identified to be MR imaging conditional, requiring no special scanning that would affect the planned research scan. No other special notations were included on the patient's written MR imaging safety screening form that was completed immediately before the scan. The patient is changed out of street clothes into the required MR imaging safe hospital gown, leaving underwear on. Because no contrast was being administered, there was no assessment by Radiology Nursing before the MR imaging. On verbal screening by the technologist, the patient again noted the presence of the penile prosthesis but disclosed nothing else of concern. The MR imaging scan was performed uneventfully. When the technologist went into the room following the scan, a lump at the waistline under the patient's gown was noted and the technologist discovered the presence of an insulin pump. The patient was removed carefully from the room, ensuring that the pump would not become a projectile. The patient examined the pump, stated that they had forgotten about it at the time of screening, and noted that it seemed to be functional. The technologist released the patient without notifying a radiologist who was immediately available and on site.

Late in the afternoon of the same day, the patient reported to the emergency department with a chief complaint of severely fluctuating blood glucoses, being intermittently markedly hyperglycemic with blood glucose in the 400s mg/dL, as well as hypoglycemic, with a reading in the low 30s mg/dL. At this time, it was recognized that the insulin pump that had been exposed to the MR imaging environment was no longer reliable. The patient was admitted to hospital to ensure medical stability while a new pump was obtained. The following day the patient was released in good condition.

Incident 4b

A 65-year-old patient was admitted for an abdomen MR imaging. The patient had been screened multiple times for metallic devices, although none were reported aside from an insulin pump on the right side of the abdomen. This was removed before scanning, leaving only the port. During the first scout, image distortion and signal loss reminiscent of metal artifact was observed on the patient's left side, which did not correspond to the location of the insulin port. The technologist queried the patient as to whether there was anything unreported during screening that was brought into the scanner room. The patient stated that there were no pumps, belts, or other devices brought into the scan room, aside from a wedding ring on the left hand. The technologist entered the scanner room, removed the ring, palpated the region around the left iliac wing, and felt nothing of concern. The technologist then ran another scout and observed that artifacts remained in the images. Technologist then inspected a recent computed tomography image of the patient and noticed metallic artifact on the lower left abdomen region, just above the left iliac wing. The technologist again queried the patient, and the patient responded that there was indeed a glucose monitor on the left side. The technologist removed the glucose monitor, and the scan was completed without further incident. The supervising technologist was alerted to the incident.

Learning points Not only are electronic implanted devices becoming more prevalent, but on-planted devices are as well. These cases highlight potentially dangerous consequences of inadvertently scanning patients with insulin pumps and associated glucose monitors. Insulin pump exposure to the MR imaging environment can alter the pump's functionality in unpredictable and hazardous ways, potentially causing life-threatening scenarios. The literature associated with the specific pump in the first incident, a Medtronic MiniMed Paradigm Revel 723 insulin pump, states that the pump should not be exposed to MR imaging or other devices that generate strong magnetic fields since the motor could be damaged and should be removed and kept outside the magnet room. It also noted that inadvertent exposure to MR imaging requires that device usage be discontinued and a 24-hour manufacturer hotline contacted. The glucose monitor in the second incident was also a concern, as it slipped by the various screening procedures undetected, and in addition to subsequent reliability concerns, could potentially cause heating or force hazards on top of the artifacts observed.

Root cause analysis of these events demonstrated a relative lack of awareness of potential severe consequences of inadvertently scanning patients with glucose monitoring equipment among technologists and radiologists. Hazard avoidance includes enhanced MR imaging safety educational efforts and augmented screening procedures. Improved screening includes updated screening forms, inclusion of device-specific information in electronic medical records, ferromagnetic-sensitive detectors, visual inspection, pat-downs, and additional verbal queries before entering the scan room. The MR imaging safety screening forms for both sites were changed to include specific questions querying the presence of insulin pumps and glucose meters, and plans were made to inquire as to whether the patient is diabetic to further identify such devices. Preliminary evidence suggests that ferromagnetic detectors can be valuable in identifying the presence of on-planted insulin pumps.

SUMMARY

As MR practices become increasingly complex, MR safety practices must continue to evolve to meet the associated challenges. It has been the intent of this article to describe real clinical scenarios that are being addressed with improved safety procedures that are in accordance with updates to the ACR guidance document on MR safe practices.[1] Sites that implement restricted access of the Zone IV doorway, a full-stop/check before entering Zone IV, screening for on-planted devices, proper separation from the bore wall, and appropriate patient gowning can help maintain a safe MR environment, benefiting patients and staff alike.

Clinics Care Points

- In the typically relatively short time that the entry door to Zone IV (MR system room) must be open (eg, for patient care), a physical "caution" barrier can help prevent unintended passage of unsafe personnel or ferromagnetic materials.
- Particularly in the acute or intraoperative environment, a full-stop/final check at the Zone IV door can help ensure unsafe items are identified and prevented from entering.
- Proper padding between the bore wall and potentially points of conductive skin to skin contact can prevent radiofrequency burns. A single bed sheet is not sufficient to prevent bore wall RF burns.

- In addition to surgically implanted devices, it is essential to recognize important MR imaging safety issues associated with "on-planted" devices, such as insulin pumps and continuous glucose monitors. There can be significant damage to the devices if exposed to MR imaging, potentially putting the patient at risk.

DISCLOSURE

The authors declare that they have no conflicts of interest or funding to disclose.

REFERENCES

1. ACR Committee on MR Safety, Greenberg TD, Hoff MN, et al. ACR guidance document on MR safe practices: updates and critical information 2019. J Magn Reson Imaging 2020;51(2):331–8.
2. Occupational Outlook Handbook: Radiologic and MRI Technologists. US Bureau of Labor Statistics. 2019. Available at: https://www.bls.gov/ooh/healthcare/radiologic-technologists.htm. Accessed March 28, 2020.
3. Cross NM, Hoff MN, Kanal KM. Avoiding MRI-related accidents: a practical approach to implementing MR safety. J Am Coll Radiol 2018;15(12):1738–44.
4. Shellock FG, Kanal E, Gilk TB. Regarding the value reported for the term "spatial gradient magnetic field" and how this information is applied to labeling of medical implants and devices. AJR Am J Roentgenol 2011;196(1):142–5.
5. Watson RE. Lessons learned from MRI safety events. Curr Radiol Rep 2015;3:37.
6. Delfino JG, Krainak DM, Flesher SA, et al. MRI-related FDA adverse event reports: a 10-yr review. Med Phys 2019;46(12):5562–71.
7. Expert Panel on MR Safety, Kanal E, Barkovich AJ, et al. ACR guidance document on MR safe practices: 2013. J Magn Reson Imaging 2013;37(3):501–30.
8. Kanal E, Barkovich AJ, Bell C, et al. ACR guidance document for safe MR practices: 2007. AJR Am J Roentgenol 2007;188(6):1447–74.
9. Kanal E, Borgstede JP, Barkovich AJ, et al. American College of Radiology White Paper on MR Safety: 2004 update and revisions. AJR Am J Roentgenol 2004;182(5):1111–4.
10. Kanal E, Borgstede JP, Barkovich AJ, et al. American College of Radiology White Paper on MR safety. AJR Am J Roentgenol 2002;178(6):1335–47.
11. Kanal E, Shaibani A. Firearm safety in the MR imaging environment. Radiology 1994;193(3):875–6.
12. Shellock FG, Crues JV. MR procedures: biologic effects, safety, and patient care. Radiology 2004;232(3):635–52.

13. Pietryga JA, Fonder MA, Rogg JM, et al. Invisible metallic microfiber in clothing presents unrecognized MRI risk for cutaneous burn. AJNR Am J Neuroradiol 2013;34(5):E47–50.

14. Bertrand A, Brunel S, Habert MO, et al. A new fire hazard for MR imaging systems: blankets-case report. Radiology 2018;286(2):568–70.

15. Federal Trade Commission. Threading Your Way Through the Labeling Requirements Under the Textile and Wool Acts. Federal Trade Commission. 2020. Available at: https://www.ftc.gov/tips-advice/business-center/guidance/threading-your-way-through-labeling-requirements-under-textile. Accessed March 20, 2020.

Statement of Ownership, Management, and Circulation
UNITED STATES POSTAL SERVICE® (All Periodicals Publications Except Requester Publications)

1. Publication Title	2. Publication Number	3. Filing Date
MAGNETIC RESONANCE IMAGING CLINICS OF NORTH AMERICA	011 – 909	9/18/2020

4. Issue Frequency	5. Number of Issues Published Annually	6. Annual Subscription Price
FEB, MAY, AUG, NOV	4	$404.00

7. Complete Mailing Address of Known Office of Publication (Not printer) (Street, city, county, state, and ZIP+4®)

ELSEVIER INC.
230 Park Avenue, Suite 800
New York, NY 10169

Contact Person
Malathi Samayan

Telephone (Include area code)
91-44-4299-4507

8. Complete Mailing Address of Headquarters or General Business Office of Publisher (Not printer)

ELSEVIER INC.
230 Park Avenue, Suite 800
New York, NY 10169

9. Full Names and Complete Mailing Addresses of Publisher, Editor, and Managing Editor (Do not leave blank)

Publisher (Name and complete mailing address)

DOLORES MELONI, ELSEVIER INC.
1600 JOHN F KENNEDY BLVD. SUITE 1800
PHILADELPHIA, PA 19103-2899

Editor (Name and complete mailing address)

JOHN VASSALLO, ELSEVIER INC.
1600 JOHN F KENNEDY BLVD. SUITE 1800
PHILADELPHIA, PA 19103-2899

Managing Editor (Name and complete mailing address)

PATRICK MANLEY, ELSEVIER INC.
1600 JOHN F KENNEDY BLVD. SUITE 1800
PHILADELPHIA, PA 19103-2899

10. Owner (Do not leave blank. If the publication is owned by a corporation, give the name and address of the corporation immediately followed by the names and addresses of all stockholders owning or holding 1 percent or more of the total amount of stock. If not owned by a corporation, give the names and addresses of the individual owners. If owned by a partnership or other unincorporated firm, give its name and address as well as those of each individual owner. If the publication is published by a nonprofit organization, give its name and address.)

Full Name	Complete Mailing Address
WHOLLY OWNED SUBSIDIARY OF REED/ELSEVIER, US HOLDINGS	1600 JOHN F KENNEDY BLVD. SUITE 1800 PHILADELPHIA, PA 19103-2899

11. Known Bondholders, Mortgagees, and Other Security Holders Owning or Holding 1 Percent or More of Total Amount of Bonds, Mortgages, or Other Securities. If none, check box → ☐ None

Full Name	Complete Mailing Address
N/A	

12. Tax Status (For completion by nonprofit organizations authorized to mail at nonprofit rates) (Check one)
The purpose, function, and nonprofit status of this organization and the exempt status for federal income tax purposes:
☒ Has Not Changed During Preceding 12 Months
☐ Has Changed During Preceding 12 Months (Publisher must submit explanation of change with this statement)

PS Form 3526, July 2014 [Page 1 of 4 (see instructions page 4)] PSN: 7530-01-000-9931 PRIVACY NOTICE: See our privacy policy on www.usps.com.

---

13. Publication Title		14. Issue Date for Circulation Data Below
MAGNETIC RESONANCE IMAGING CLINICS OF NORTH AMERICA		MAY 2020

15. Extent and Nature of Circulation			Average No. Copies Each Issue During Preceding 12 Months	No. Copies of Single Issue Published Nearest to Filing Date
a. Total Number of Copies (Net press run)			363	322
b. Paid Circulation (By Mail and Outside the Mail)	(1)	Mailed Outside-County Paid Subscriptions Stated on PS Form 3541 (Include paid distribution above nominal rate, advertiser's proof copies, and exchange copies)	280	250
	(2)	Mailed In-County Paid Subscriptions Stated on PS Form 3541 (Include paid distribution above nominal rate, advertiser's proof copies, and exchange copies)	0	0
	(3)	Paid Distribution Outside the Mails Including Sales Through Dealers and Carriers, Street Vendors, Counter Sales, and Other Paid Distribution Outside USPS®	66	59
	(4)	Paid Distribution by Other Classes of Mail Through the USPS (e.g. First-Class Mail®)	0	0
c. Total Paid Distribution (Sum of 15b (1), (2), (3), and (4))			346	309
d. Free or Nominal Rate Distribution (By Mail and Outside the Mail)	(1)	Free or Nominal Rate Outside-County Copies included on PS Form 3541	17	13
	(2)	Free or Nominal Rate In-County Copies Included on PS Form 3541	0	0
	(3)	Free or Nominal Rate Copies Mailed at Other Classes Through the USPS (e.g. First-Class Mail)	0	0
	(4)	Free or Nominal Rate Distribution Outside the Mail (Carriers or other means)	0	0
e. Total Free or Nominal Rate Distribution (Sum of 15d (1), (2), (3) and (4))			17	13
f. Total Distribution (Sum of 15c and 15e)			363	322
g. Copies not Distributed (See instructions to Publishers #4 (page #3))			0	0
h. Total (Sum of 15f and g)			363	322
i. Percent Paid (15c divided by 15f times 100)			95.31%	95.96%

* If you are claiming electronic copies, go to line 16 on page 3. If you are not claiming electronic copies, skip to line 17 on page 3.

16. Electronic Copy Circulation	Average No. Copies Each Issue During Preceding 12 Months	No. Copies of Single Issue Published Nearest to Filing Date
a. Paid Electronic Copies		
b. Total Paid Print Copies (Line 15c) + Paid Electronic Copies (Line 16a)		
c. Total Print Distribution (Line 15f) + Paid Electronic Copies (Line 16a)		
d. Percent Paid (Both Print & Electronic Copies) (16b divided by 16c × 100)		

☒ I certify that 50% of all my distributed copies (electronic and print) are paid above a nominal price.

17. Publication of Statement of Ownership
☒ If the publication is a general publication, publication of this statement is required. Will be printed in the NOVEMBER 2020 issue of this publication. ☐ Publication not required.

18. Signature and Title of Editor, Publisher, Business Manager, or Owner

Malathi Samayan - Distribution Controller

Malathi Samayan   Date 9/18/2020

I certify that all information furnished on this form is true and complete. I understand that anyone who furnishes false or misleading information on this form or who omits material or information requested on the form may be subject to criminal sanctions (including fines and imprisonment) and/or civil sanctions (including civil penalties).

PS Form 3526, July 2014 (Page 3 of 4) PRIVACY NOTICE: See our privacy policy on www.usps.com

Moving?

Make sure your subscription moves with you!

To notify us of your new address, find your **Clinics Account Number** (located on your mailing label above your name), and contact customer service at:

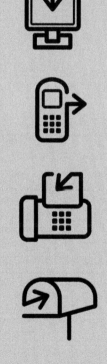

Email: **journalscustomerservice-usa@elsevier.com**

800-654-2452 (subscribers in the U.S. & Canada)
314-447-8871 (subscribers outside of the U.S. & Canada)

Fax number: **314-447-8029**

Elsevier Health Sciences Division
Subscription Customer Service
3251 Riverport Lane
Maryland Heights, MO 63043

*To ensure uninterrupted delivery of your subscription, please notify us at least 4 weeks in advance of move.

Printed and bound by CPI Group (UK) Ltd, Croydon, CR0 4YY

08/05/2025

01864692-0008